GET
LAID

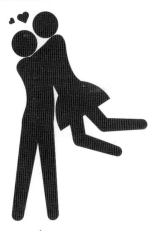

D0753818

GET LAID

AMANDA HUNTER

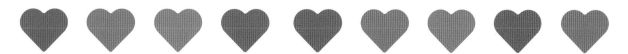

weldon**owen**

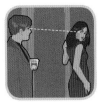

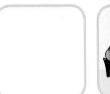

how to
use this
book

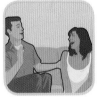

dating tips

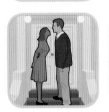

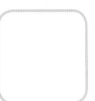

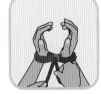

flirty
games

♥ bond

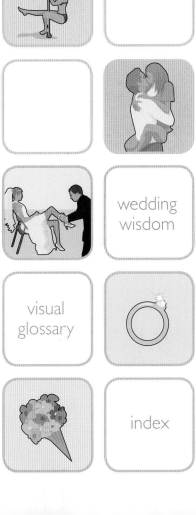
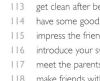
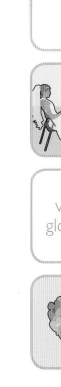
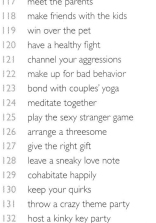

steamy moves

wedding wisdom

visual glossary

index

a note from amanda

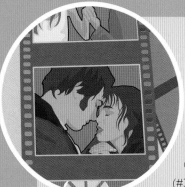

48 match the kiss to the mood

As a dating and relationships writer, I've advised readers on everything from the romantic to the raunchy—from the perfect kiss (#48) to the perfect lap dance (#69). When I sat down to write this book, I drew from that experience as well as my personal interest in things like picking up cute guys at dog parks (#38), sassy ways to flirt (#35), and what to do once you get him home (#87) . . . as well a few varsity moves (#97)! Throughout the process, I learned a few awesome things, including how to play with candles (#79), a way to make duct tape sexy (#101), and what to do with that ottoman (#89). I'm not sure I'm going to be throwing a '70s-style key party (#132) or getting it on with the pool boy (#96) any time soon but hey, it can't hurt to know how, just in case!

38 find puppy love at a dog park

69 surprise with a lap dance

AMANDA is the psuedonym of a relationships author and columnist who's given expert advice on many subjects including dating (#47), decoding body language (#24), and staying safe (#26). She recently married her longtime sweetheart (#148), whom she did not, in fact, meet on a bus (#23). She did, however, do a wonderful job of packing for the honeymoon (#149). And she's not using her real name because she doesn't want her mother to know she ties a mean Texas handcuff (#98).

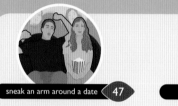

sneak an arm around a date 47

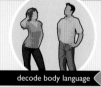

decode body language 24

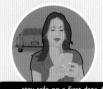

stay safe on a first date 26

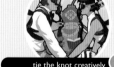
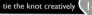

tie the knot creatively 148

get carried away on the bus 23

fold her clothes for travel 149

how to use this book

In the pages that follow, virtually every piece of essential information is presented graphically. In most cases the pictures do, indeed, tell the whole story. In some cases though, you'll need a little extra information to get it done right. Here's how we present those facts.

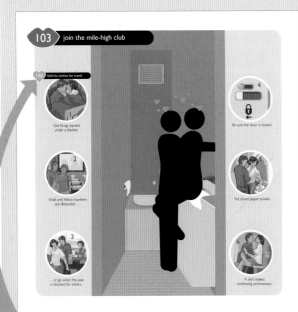

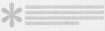

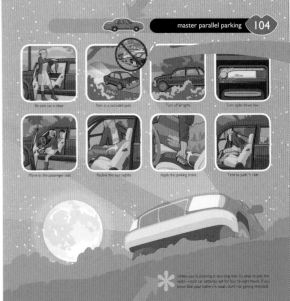

CROSS-REFERENCES When one thing just leads to another, we'll point it out. Follow the links for related or interesting information.

150 fold his clothes for travel

MORE INFORMATION Follow the * symbol to learn more about the how and why of the given step.

TOOLS Everything you'll need to perform an activity appears in the toolbars. Having a hard time deciphering an item? Turn to the tools glossary in the back of the book.

ZOOMS These little circles zoom in on a step's important details, or depict the step's crucial "don'ts."

ICON GUIDE Throughout the book, handy icons show you just how it's done. Here are the icons you'll encounter.

 Check out the timer to learn how much time a relatively short task takes.

 The calendar shows how many days, weeks, or months an activity requires.

 Look to the thermometer to learn the temperature needed for a given action.

 Repeat the depicted action the designated number of times.

 Just how hot, you ask? Cook over low, medium, or high heat, respectively.

A NOTE TO READERS The depictions in this book are presented for entertainment value only. Please keep the following in mind:

- RISKY ACTIVITIES Certain activities in this book are not just risky but downright nutty. Before attempting any new activity, make sure you are aware of your own limitations and have adequately researched all applicable risks.

- PROFESSIONAL ADVICE While every item has been carefully researched, this book is not intended to replace professional advice or training of a medical, culinary, sartorial, romantic, athletic, or therapeutic nature—or any other professional advice, for that matter.

- PHYSICAL AND HEALTH-RELATED ACTIVITIES Be sure to consult a physician before attempting any activity involving physical exertion, particularly if you have a condition that could impair or limit your ability to engage in such an activity. Or if you don't want to look silly (see #68).

- ADULT CONTENT The activities in this book are intended for adults only. Some of them are probably unwise even for adults; use your common sense and discretion (if, for instance, you plan to attempt #99).

- BREAKING THE LAW The information in this book should not be used to break any applicable law or regulation. In other words, just don't even try #103.

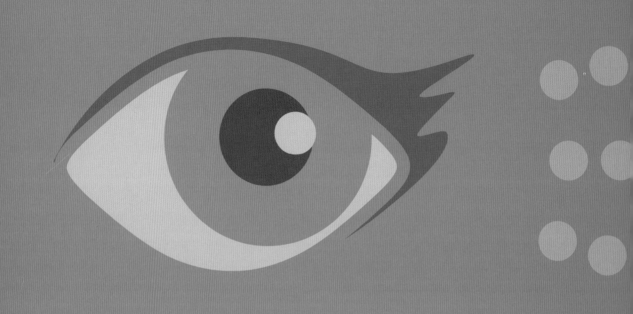

flirt

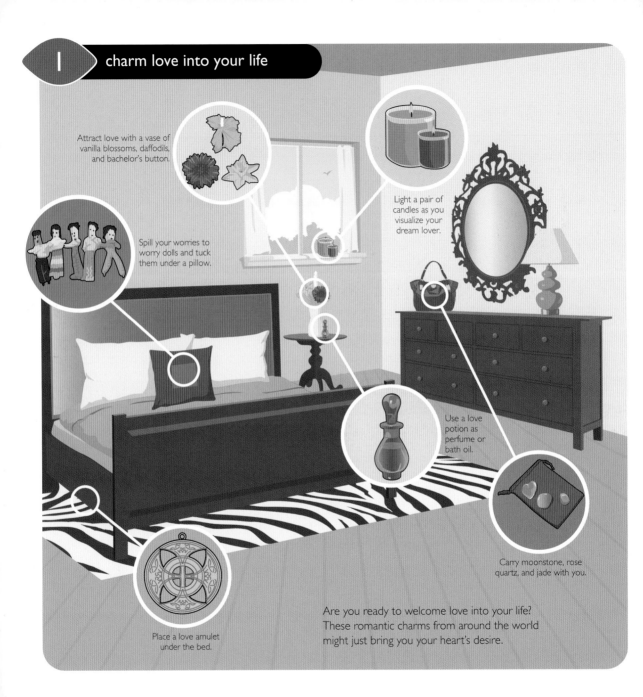

Attract love with a vase of vanilla blossoms, daffodils, and bachelor's button.

Light a pair of candles as you visualize your dream lover.

Spill your worries to worry dolls and tuck them under a pillow.

Use a love potion as perfume or bath oil.

Carry moonstone, rose quartz, and jade with you.

Place a love amulet under the bed.

Are you ready to welcome love into your life? These romantic charms from around the world might just bring you your heart's desire.

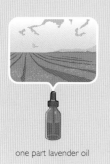 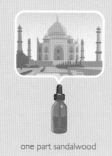 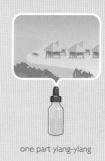 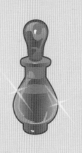

one part lavender oil   one part sandalwood   one part ylang-ylang

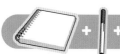 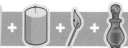

bathe your way to love 3

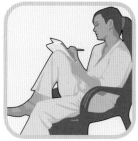

Describe your perfect lover.

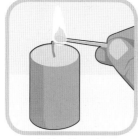

Light a pink candle.

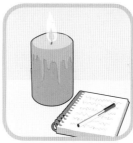

Place the list by the candle.

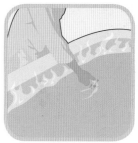

Draw a warm bath.

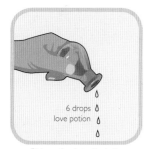

Drip potion into the bath.

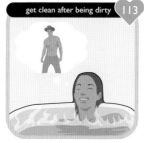

get clean after being dirty 113

Soak, visualizing your lover.

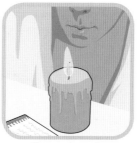

Blow out the candle.

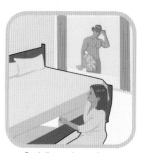

Stash list; await your lover.

6 drops
love potion

4 look flirty at the club

Hit the club feeling sexy, not skanky. Your confidence will work like a magnet on the dance floor.

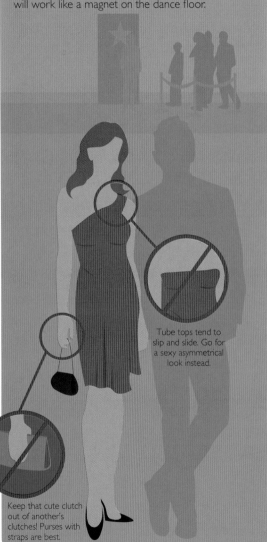

Tube tops tend to slip and slide. Go for a sexy asymmetrical look instead.

Keep that cute clutch out of another's clutches! Purses with straps are best.

5 go cozy-chic on movie night

Movie night is a good chance to show off your laid-back charms with a casually stylish outfit.

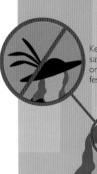

Keep a low profile, and save your dramatic hat or hairdo for a more festive occasion.

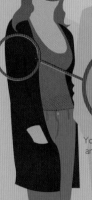

You're hot, but theaters are cold. Bring a warm, flattering sweater.

93 shoot a sexy home movie

Strike a perfect balance between playful and elegant by pairing something classic with a splash of color.

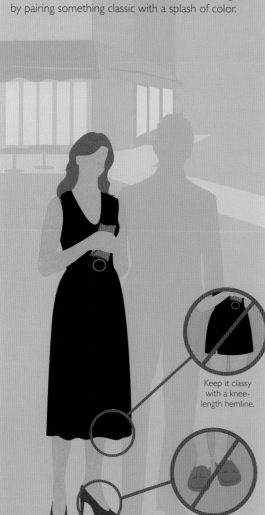

Keep it classy with a knee-length hemline.

Show off your stems with a pair of pumps.

When dating alfresco, come prepared with comfy, cute layers and a bag of picnic supplies.

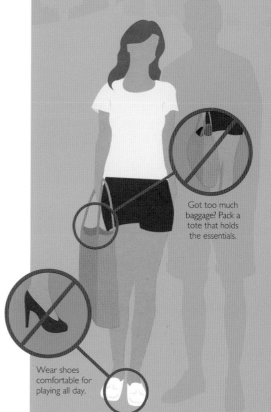

Got too much baggage? Pack a tote that holds the essentials.

Wear shoes comfortable for playing all day.

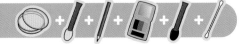

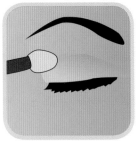

Apply primer to eyelid.

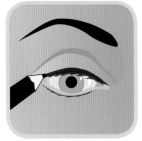

Line top lid with dark pencil.

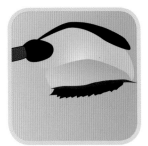

Highlight entire brow bone.

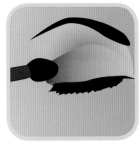

Add a medium color.

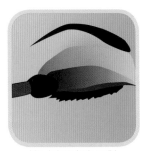

Use darkest shade on lid.

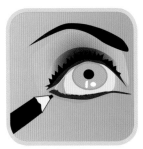

Line beneath eye.

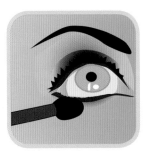

Add a swipe of eyeshadow.

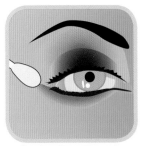

Smudge with a cotton swab.

9 give yourself a sultry pout

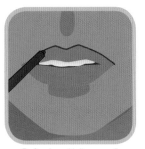

Define lips with liner pencil.

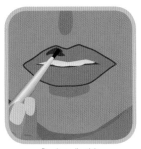

Brush on lipstick.

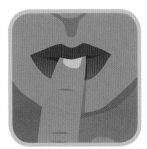

Suck finger to blot.

48 match the kiss to the mood

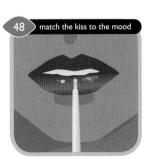

Dab clear gloss in center.

roll up luscious waves 10

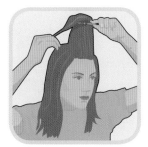

Separate hair into sections.

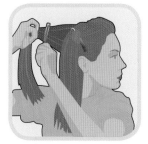

Clip sections as needed.

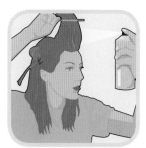

Mist with hairspray; comb.

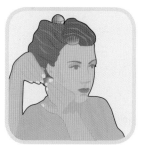

Wrap hair around curlers.

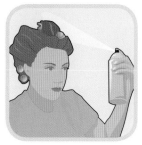

Mist with hairspray.

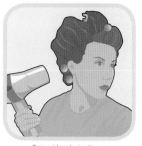

Set with a hair dryer.

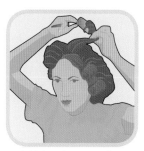

Let hair cool; remove rollers.

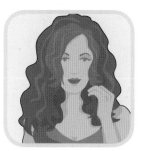

Comb with fingers to style.

walk like a diva in heels 11

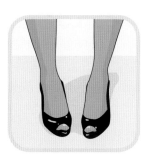

Start with feet turned in.

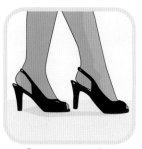

Put your toe down first.

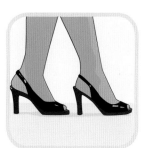

Land heel in front of toe.

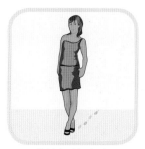

Hold shoulders back.

12 tame a unibrow

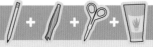

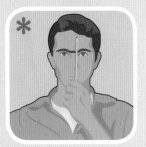

Find the best brow shape.

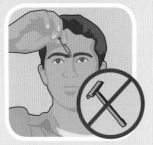

Pluck slowly and carefully.

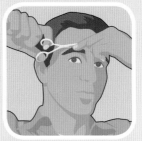

Trim long hairs with scissors.

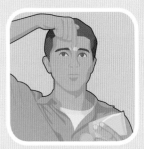

Soothe skin with aloe.

✳ Looking like a Neanderthal is so 400,000 years ago. Find the endpoints of your soon-to-be-dual brows by holding a pencil alongside your nose. Pluck on the bridge side of the pencil.

14 knot a bow tie

1

2

3

4

5

6

7

8

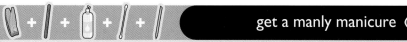

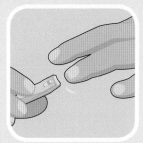

Clip straight across.

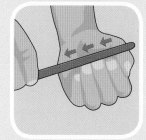

File in one direction.

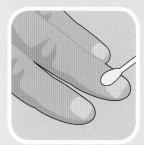

Moisturize cuticles.

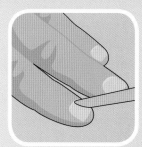

Gently push back cuticles.

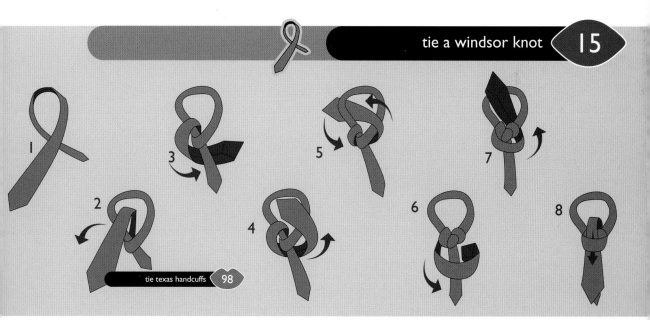

tie texas handcuffs 98

16   look like a stud at the club

Want to make her VIP list? You can't go wrong when sporting a sleek but relaxed outfit.

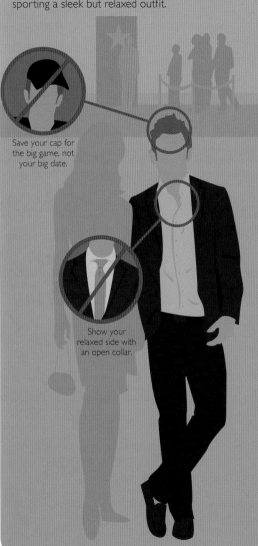

Save your cap for the big game, not your big date.

Show your relaxed side with an open collar.

17   master a movie-date look

Nicely cut jeans and a sharp sweater show her that you can go casual without looking clueless.

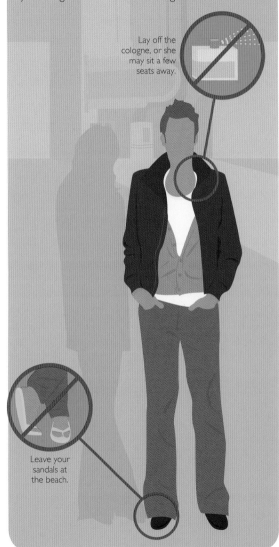

Lay off the cologne, or she may sit a few seats away.

Leave your sandals at the beach.

You've got a table at a fancy hot spot—your look should say "filet mignon," not "country-fried steak."

Even if she loves your beard, give it a trim before heading to a swanky restaurant.

Tonight's kind of a big deal. Wear a nice button-down.

Even if you're hoping for a roll in the bushes later on, start with clean, wrinkle-free clothes.

master the art of manscaping 71

No shirt, no shoes, no second date! Keep your shirt on.

Who wears short-shorts? A man who ends up going home alone.

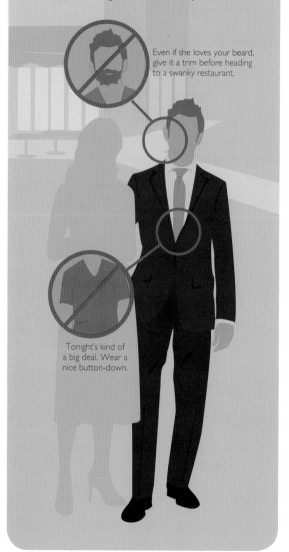

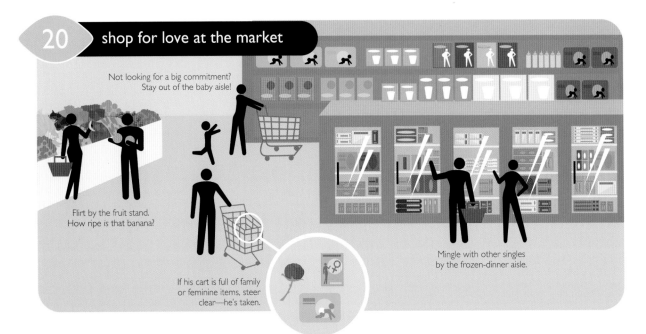

20 shop for love at the market

Not looking for a big commitment? Stay out of the baby aisle!

Flirt by the fruit stand. How ripe *is* that banana?

If his cart is full of family or feminine items, steer clear—he's taken.

Mingle with other singles by the frozen-dinner aisle.

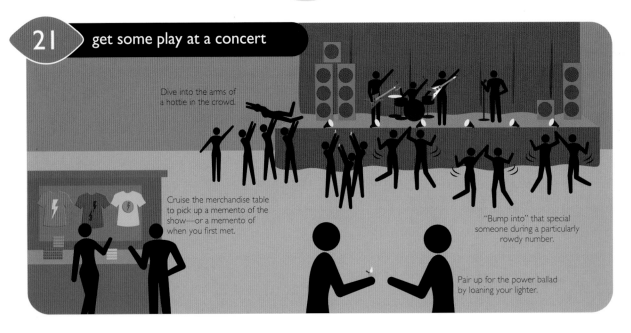

21 get some play at a concert

Dive into the arms of a hottie in the crowd.

Cruise the merchandise table to pick up a memento of the show—or a memento of when you first met.

"Bump into" that special someone during a particularly rowdy number.

Pair up for the power ballad by loaning your lighter.

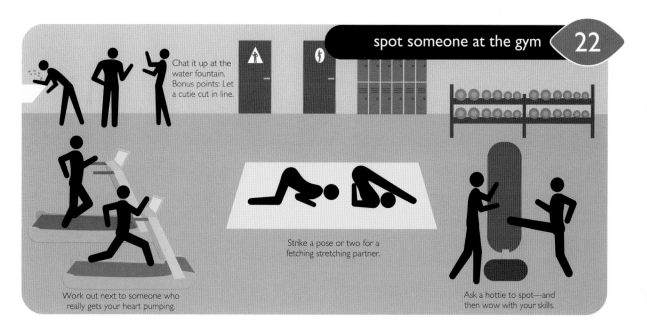

Chat it up at the water fountain. Bonus points: Let a cutie cut in line.

Strike a pose or two for a fetching stretching partner.

Work out next to someone who really gets your heart pumping.

Ask a hottie to spot—and then wow with your skills.

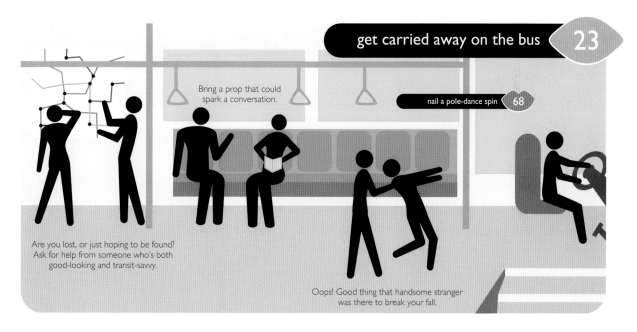

Bring a prop that could spark a conversation.

nail a pole-dance spin 68

Are you lost, or just hoping to be found? Ask for help from someone who's both good-looking and transit-savvy.

Oops! Good thing that handsome stranger was there to break your fall.

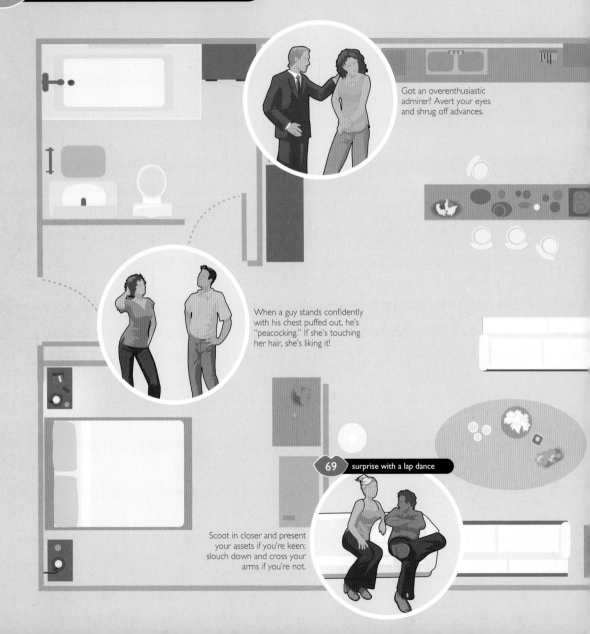

Got an overenthusiastic admirer? Avert your eyes and shrug off advances.

When a guy stands confidently with his chest puffed out, he's "peacocking." If she's touching her hair, she's liking it!

69 surprise with a lap dance

Scoot in closer and present your assets if you're keen; slouch down and cross your arms if you're not.

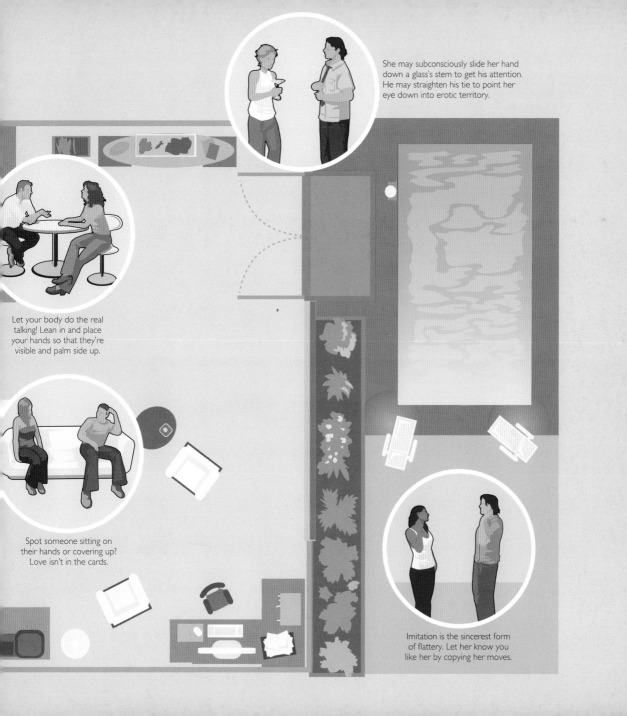

She may subconsciously slide her hand down a glass's stem to get his attention. He may straighten his tie to point her eye down into erotic territory.

Let your body do the real talking! Lean in and place your hands so that they're visible and palm side up.

Spot someone sitting on their hands or covering up? Love isn't in the cards.

Imitation is the sincerest form of flattery. Let her know you like her by copying her moves.

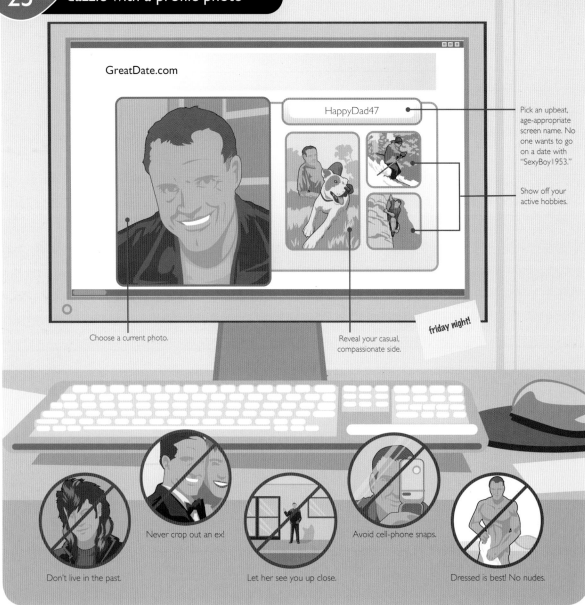

GreatDate.com

HappyDad47

Pick an upbeat, age-appropriate screen name. No one wants to go on a date with "SexyBoy1953."

Show off your active hobbies.

friday night!

Choose a current photo.

Reveal your casual, compassionate side.

Don't live in the past.

Never crop out an ex!

Let her see you up close.

Avoid cell-phone snaps.

Dressed is best! No nudes.

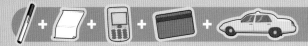
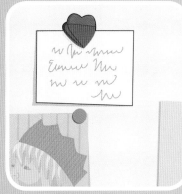

Leave a note saying where you'll be.

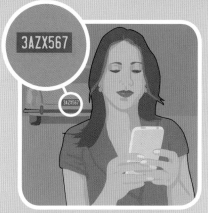

Text your friends his license-plate number.

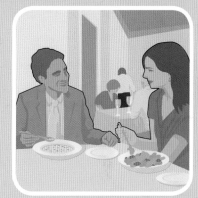

Meet in a public place.

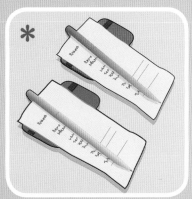

Split the check.

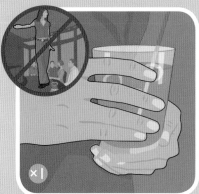

Go easy on the booze.

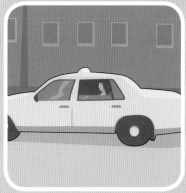

Plan your own ride home.

 Who should pay? Ultimately, the check should be settled so that everyone feels comfortable and respected. If either party seems like an ungracious freeloader, or pays the bill and expects something in return, it's a sign to end the date.

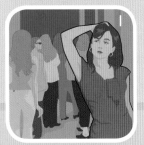

Wait for the crowd to pass.

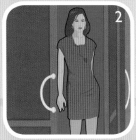

Enter with confidence.

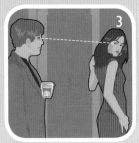

Make eye contact; smile.

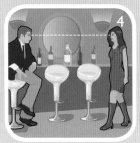

Identify a destination.

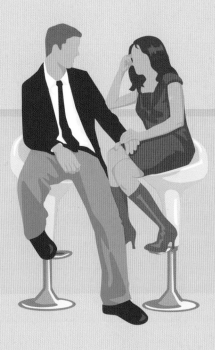

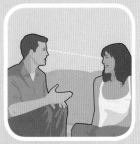

Maintain eye contact.

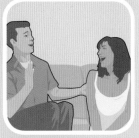

Crack jokes.

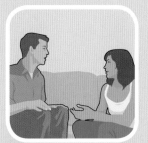

Ask thoughtful questions.

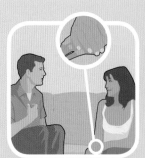

Sit calmly, don't fidget.

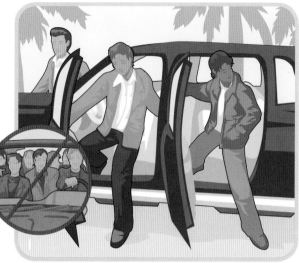

Go out with a small number of friends.

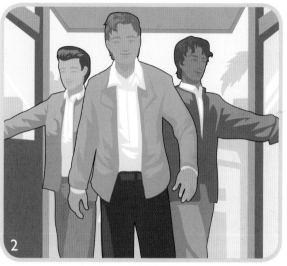

Establish yourself as the alpha male.

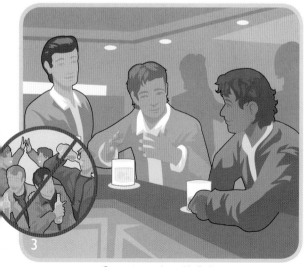

Comport yourselves with dignity.

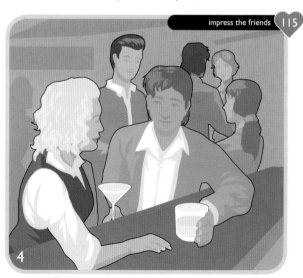

Forge on alone when you meet someone promising.

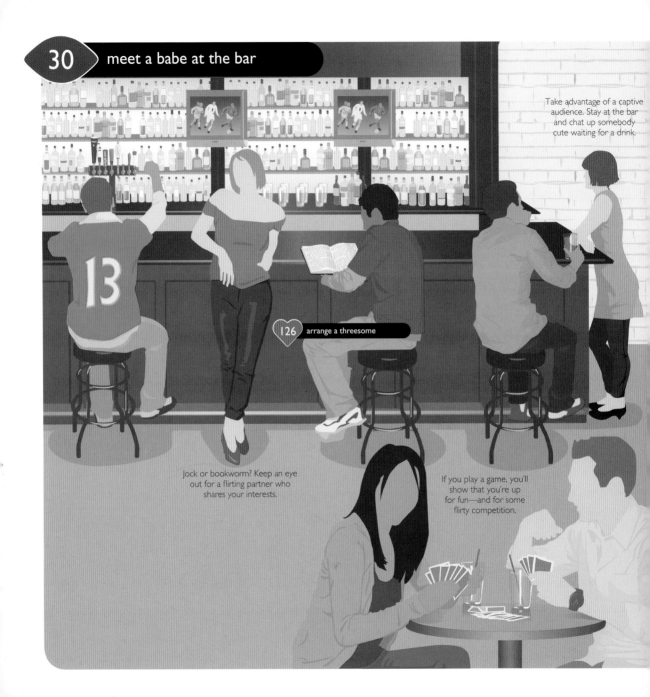

Take advantage of a captive audience. Stay at the bar and chat up somebody cute waiting for a drink.

126 arrange a threesome

Jock or bookworm? Keep an eye out for a flirting partner who shares your interests.

If you play a game, you'll show that you're up for fun—and for some flirty competition.

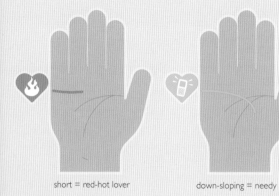

short = red-hot lover

down-sloping = needy

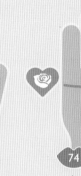

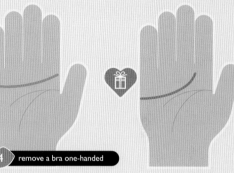

74 remove a bra one-handed

long = romantic

up-sloping = giving

tie a sexy cherry-stem knot 35

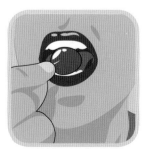

Eat cherry; save stem.

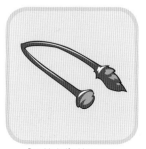

Bend in half with tongue.

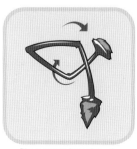

Bite a corner, loop through.

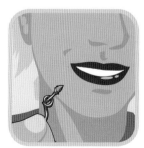

Tighten with teeth; display.

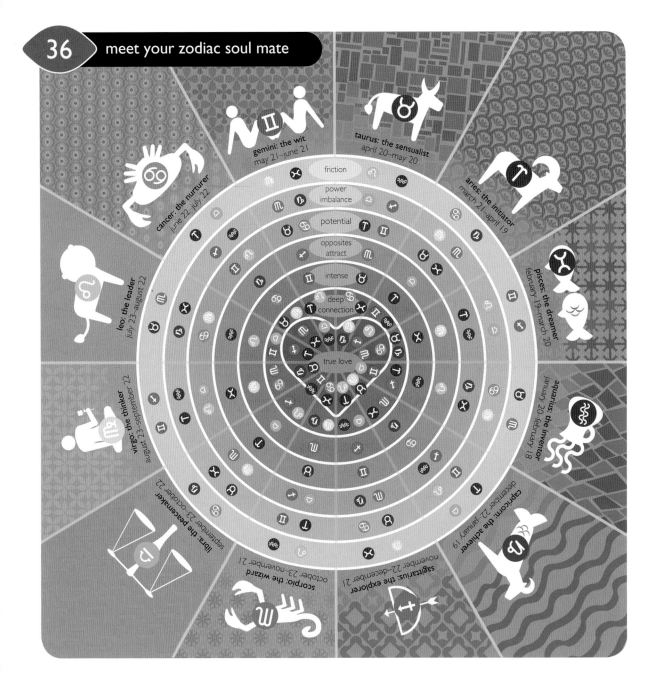

gemini: the wit
may 21–june 21

taurus: the sensualist
april 20–may 20

cancer: the nurturer
june 22–july 22

aries: the initiator
march 21–april 19

leo: the leader
july 23–august 22

pisces: the dreamer
february 19–march 20

virgo: the thinker
august 23–september 22

aquarius: the inventor
january 20–february 18

libra: the peacemaker
september 23–october 22

capricorn: the achiever
december 22–january 19

scorpio: the wizard
october 23–november 21

sagittarius: the explorer
november 22–december 21

friction

power imbalance

potential

opposites attract

intense

deep connection

true love

To learn your Chinese zodiac sign, find the year of your birth below. (If you were born early in the year, check a calendar to see if the Chinese New Year fell after your birthday.) Your best love matches are listed in the same column as your sign.

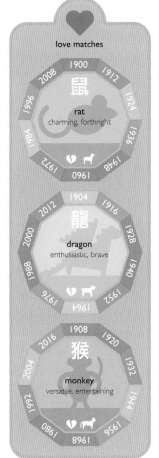

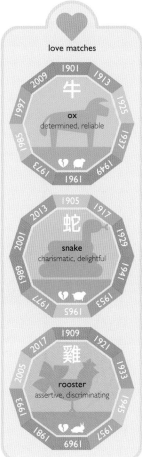

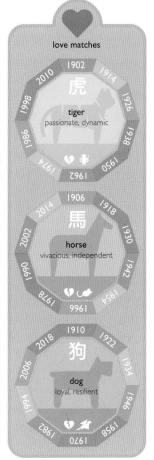

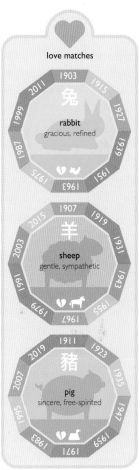

love matches

love matches

love matches

love matches

鼠
rat
charming, forthright
1900 1912 1924 1936 1948 1960 1972 1984 1996 2008

牛
ox
determined, reliable
1901 1913 1925 1937 1949 1961 1973 1985 1997 2009

虎
tiger
passionate, dynamic
1902 1914 1926 1938 1950 1962 1974 1986 1998 2010

兔
rabbit
gracious, refined
1903 1915 1927 1939 1951 1963 1975 1987 1999 2011

龍
dragon
enthusiastic, brave
1904 1916 1928 1940 1952 1964 1976 1988 2000 2012

蛇
snake
charismatic, delightful
1905 1917 1929 1941 1953 1965 1977 1989 2001 2013

馬
horse
vivacious, independent
1906 1918 1930 1942 1954 1966 1978 1990 2002 2014

羊
sheep
gentle, sympathetic
1907 1919 1931 1943 1955 1967 1979 1991 2003 2015

猴
monkey
versatile, entertaining
1908 1920 1932 1944 1956 1968 1980 1992 2004 2016

雞
rooster
assertive, discriminating
1909 1921 1933 1945 1957 1969 1981 1993 2005 2017

狗
dog
loyal, resilient
1910 1922 1934 1946 1958 1970 1982 1994 2006 2018

豬
pig
sincere, free-spirited
1911 1923 1935 1947 1959 1971 1983 1995 2007 2019

Each animal sign and birth year is paired with a natural element. Match the colors at right to the animals and birth years of your love connections for a deeper understanding.

earth
generous, cooperative

fire
animated, restless

wood
disciplined, tenacious

metal
unyielding, reserved

water
secretive, creative

When you're cruising the dog park, you'll run into many different breeds of dogs—and many different breeds of possible dates! Here's what the pooch says about the owner.

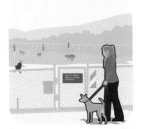

Go at busy times.

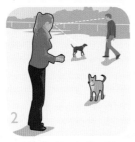

2

Spot the right dog (owner).

91 play with grown-up toys

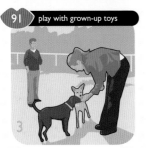

3

Share your toys.

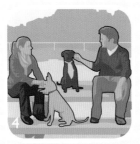

4

Chat up the hot owner.

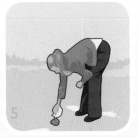

5

Respect dog-park etiquette.

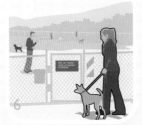

6

Follow a routine.

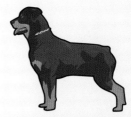

assertive, serious, dominant

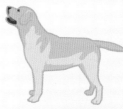

happy, fun, loves kids

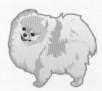

playful, high-maintenance (or walking his girlfriend's dog!)

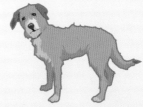

compassionate, loyal, loving

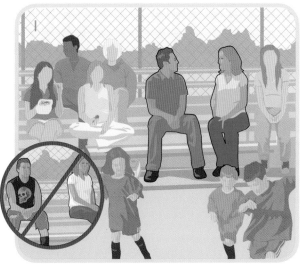

Dress to impress.

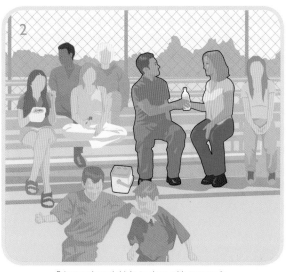

Bring snacks and drinks to share with your crush.

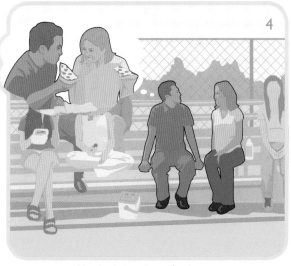

Get excited about the game, but not too excited.

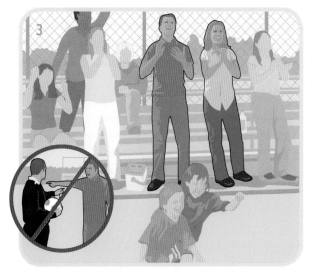

Make plans to have dinner after the game.

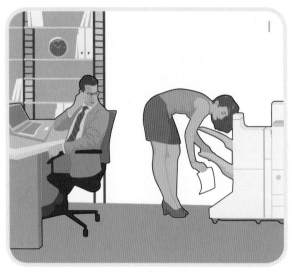

Make yourself noticeable.

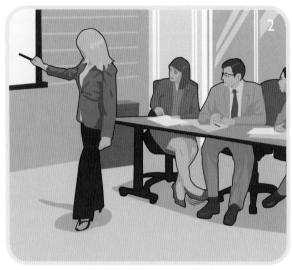

Play footsie during boring meetings.

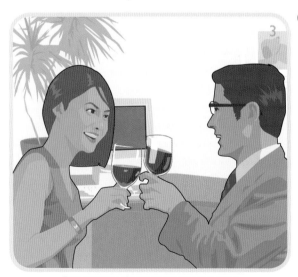

Take advantage of happy hour and "working late."

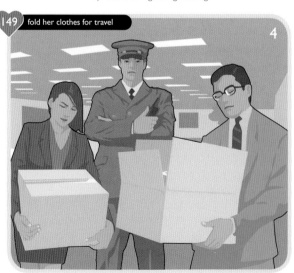

149   fold her clothes for travel

Know the company policy on intraoffice dating.

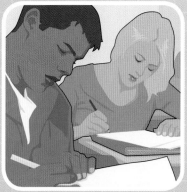
Sit close to your crush.

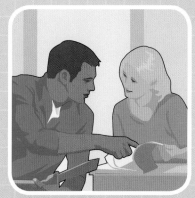
Discuss interesting ideas in class.

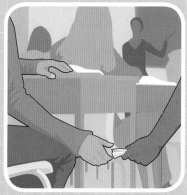
Pass notes during lecture.

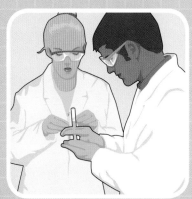
Team up on projects.

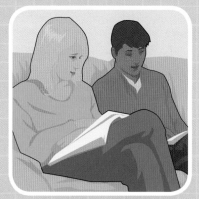
Study together outside of school.

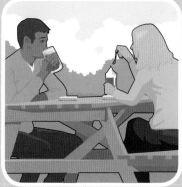
Celebrate after an exam.

launch love with a paper plane

 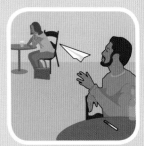

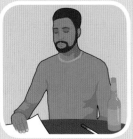

Find a napkin.

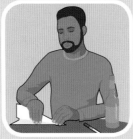

Fold into a paper airplane.

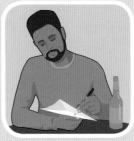

Write a witty note.

Watch it soar.

twist a napkin rose

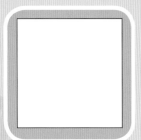

Unfold a napkin.

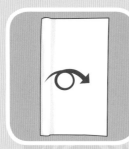

Roll into a tube.

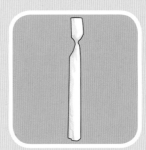

Pinch to create a bud.

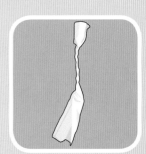

Tightly twist to make a stem.

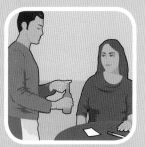

Buy a bottled beer.

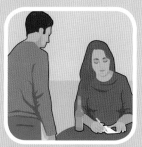

Jot an enticing note.

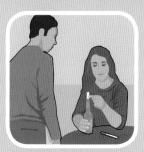

Roll; slip into bottle.

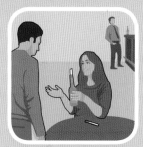

Have it hand delivered.

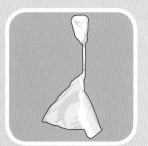

Unroll a triangle shape.

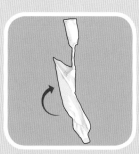

Pull up to make a leaf.

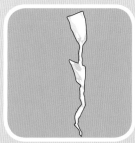

Continue twisting the stem.

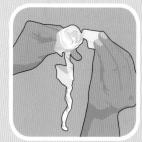

Slyly slide a note inside.

What to bring on that all-important first date?
The basics should fit in a purse or pocket, and
the goal is to look nice, smell better, and be safe.

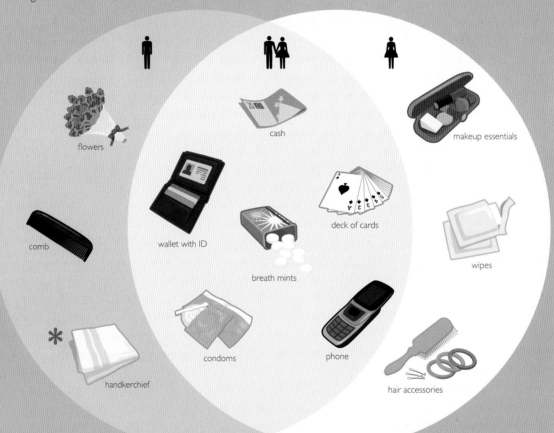

flowers

cash

makeup essentials

comb

wallet with ID

deck of cards

breath mints

wipes

* handkerchief

condoms

phone

hair accessories

 Who carries a handkerchief these days? Gentlemen who
want to impress! Use it to mop up her spilled drink, clean
off a dusty bus seat, or dab a tear from your eye.

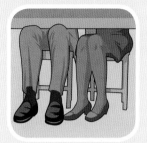

Assess interest with a tap.

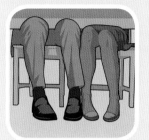

Move in closer.

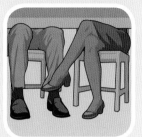

Coyly rub and lock ankles.

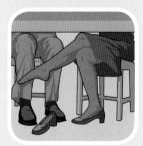

Shed a shoe.

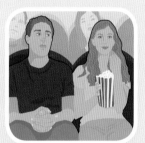

Wait until she's at ease.

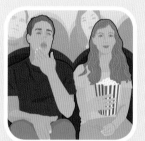

Begin the classic yawn.

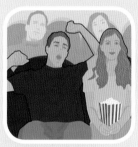

Stretch, raising your arm.

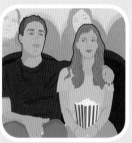

Land it.

Is your relationship a romantic comedy or a torrid tale? As the story unspools, your kiss will reflect the intensity of your passion.

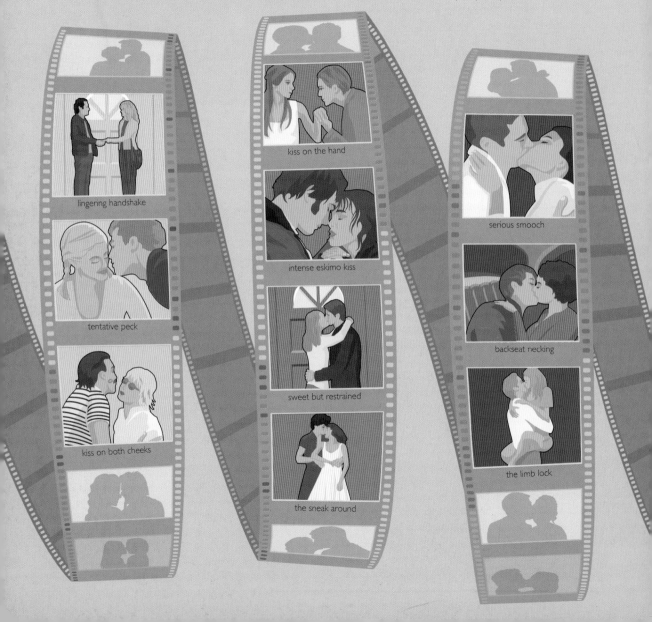

lingering handshake

tentative peck

kiss on both cheeks

kiss on the hand

intense eskimo kiss

sweet but restrained

the sneak around

serious smooch

backseat necking

the limb lock

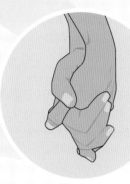

romantic feelings

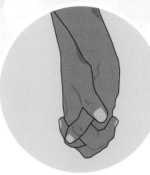

deeper intimacy

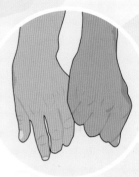

playful and silly

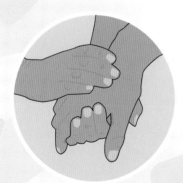

old-fashioned and sweet

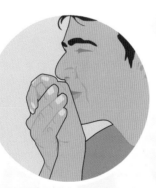

increasing affection

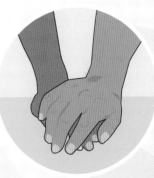

feeling protective

Get swept up in a European classic. Rotate slightly after every three beats for that whirling effect.

Hey, daddy-o! This quick-stepped dance keeps you on the balls of your feet. Kicks and turns are welcome.

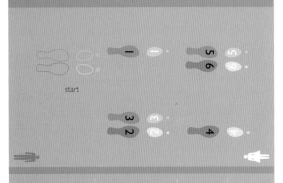

start

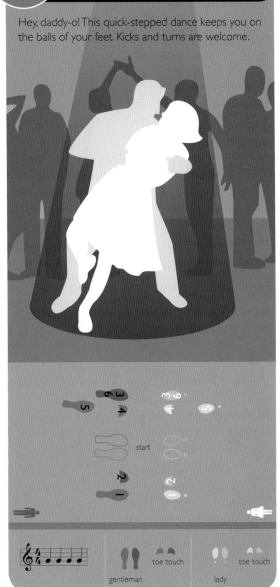

start

3/4 ♩♩♩ emphasis	path across dance floor	gentleman	lady

4/4 ♩♩♩♩	gentleman	toe touch	lady	toe touch

For a smoldering tango, take the first two steps slow, the next two quick, and the last superslow and sexy.

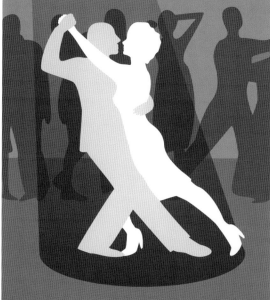

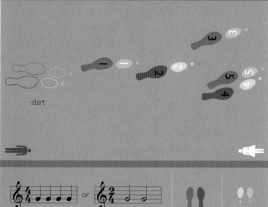

start

gentleman

lady

This feisty dance is all about the hips. You can do these steps in any direction—even while spinning.

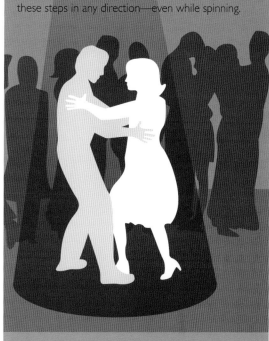

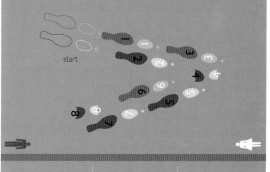

start

toe touch

gentleman

toe touch

lady

toe touch

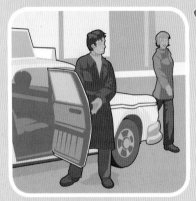

Open the car door for her.

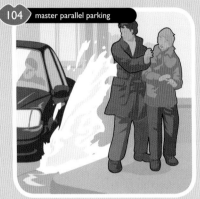

104 master parallel parking

Walk on the street side.

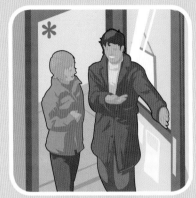

Hold the door for her.

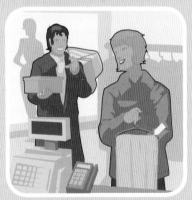

Carry her bags.

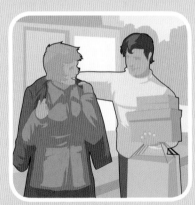

Offer your coat.

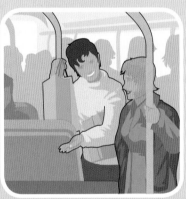

Make sure she has a seat.

Not every woman wants to be treated like a princess.
If the lady asks you to ease up on the chivalry, be a
true gentleman—oblige her gracefully.

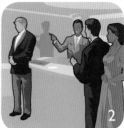

Look like you belong.

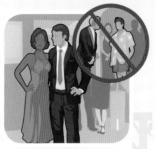

Figure out who's in charge.

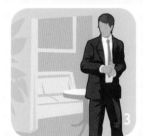

Fold the bill discreetly.

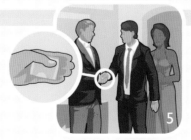

Approach with confidence.

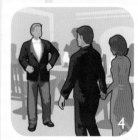

Transfer with a handshake.

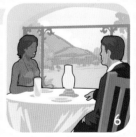

Enjoy a great table.

eat elegantly on a dinner date

Variety is the spice of life. Order a spread of tapas plates, then compare favorites.

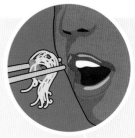

Show off your chopstick chops by eating stir-fry with ease.

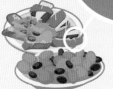

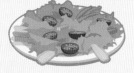

salad

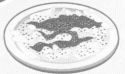

small plates

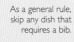

bite-size pasta

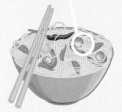

stir-fried noodles

---

avoid turn-off dishes

As a general rule, skip any dish that requires a bib.

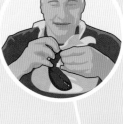

Don't order a stinky dish—unless your date is ordering it, too.

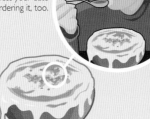

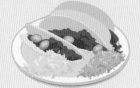

messy tacos

french onion soup

beans

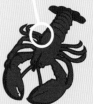

shellfish

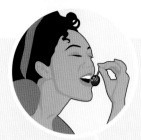

Make a sensual display of eating berries and fruits.

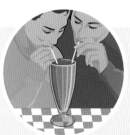

A milkshake is a great excuse to get superclose.

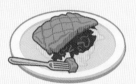

easy-to-cut meat

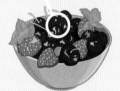

cherries and strawberries

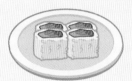

small sushi rolls

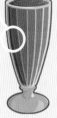

milkshake

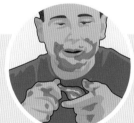

Chicken wings are labor-intensive and messy.

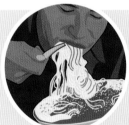

Slurping is rarely sexy. Steer clear of long noodles.

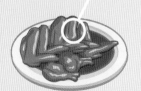

chicken wings

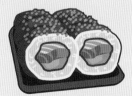

large sushi rolls

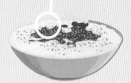

spaghetti

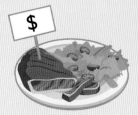

$

expensive steak

58 give a polite kiss-off

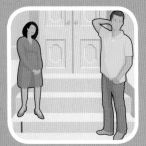
Shy away from contact.

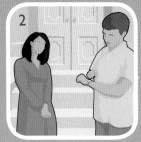
Say it's getting late.

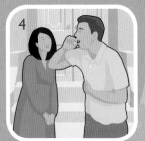
Hint at other plans.

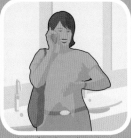
Feign sickness.

59 cut a bad date short

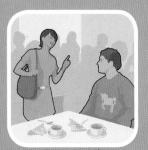
Excuse yourself.

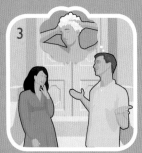
Ask a friend to call you back.

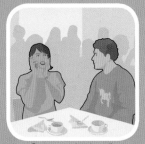
Return; receive the call.

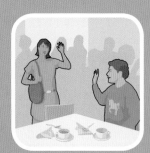
Claim an emergency. Leave.

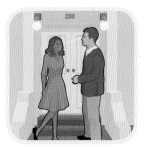

Stand close; gaze into eyes.

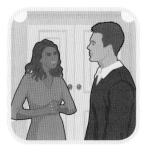

Say you had a good time.

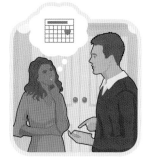

Plan your next date.

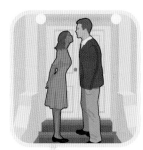

Hug (or kiss!) goodnight.

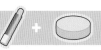

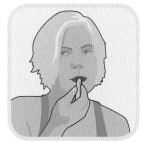

Make your lips kissable.

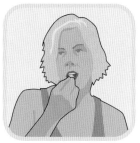

Keep your breath fresh!

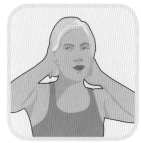

Tame any unruly hair.

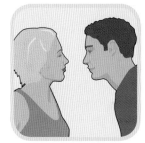

Make eye contact; lean in.

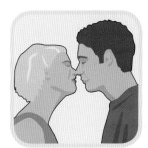

Tilt; close your eyes.

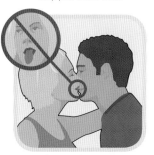

Let your lips meet.

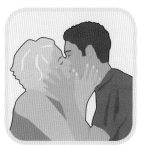

Get your hands involved.

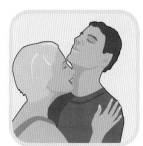

Explore new territory.

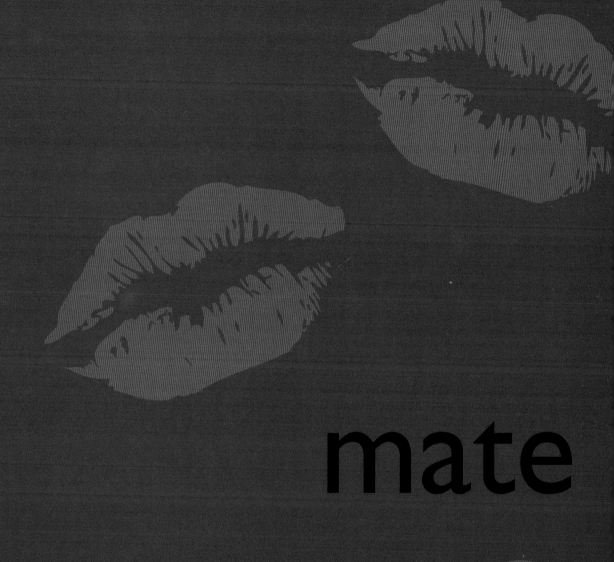

mate

You've met that special someone and invited him or her back to your love nest. To keep your dream date from turning into a nightmare, stash that pile of dirty dishes—and the even dirtier magazines.

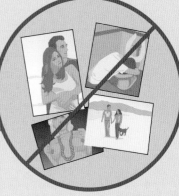

The photos you choose to display say a lot about you.

Display conversation starters that show off your interests.

Queue up a few hours of classy slow jams ahead of time.

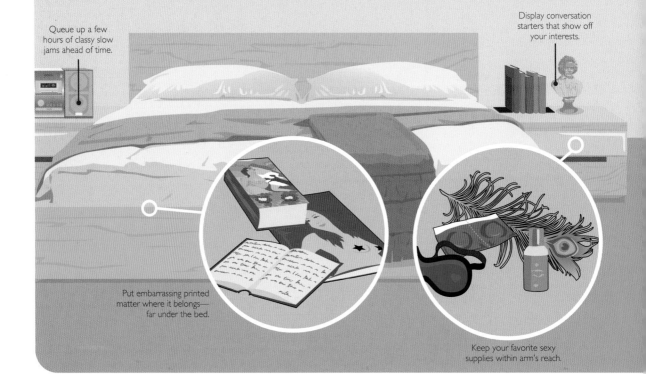

Put embarrassing printed matter where it belongs—far under the bed.

Keep your favorite sexy supplies within arm's reach.

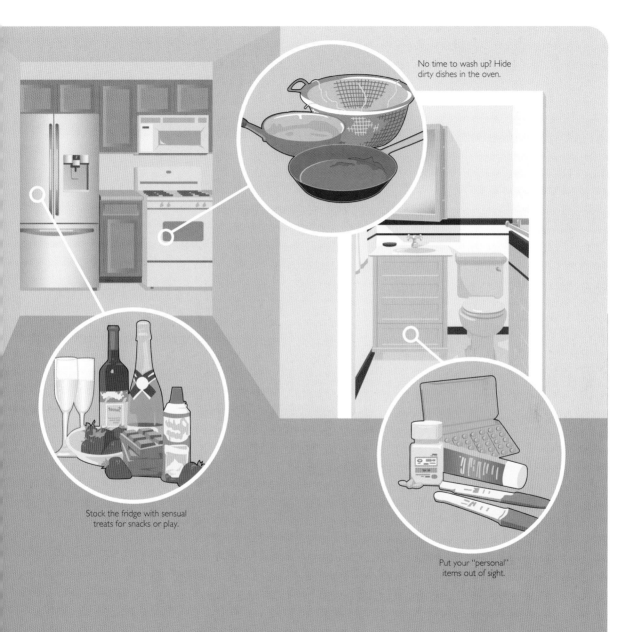

No time to wash up? Hide dirty dishes in the oven.

Stock the fridge with sensual treats for snacks or play.

Put your "personal" items out of sight.

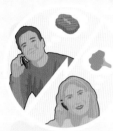

Clear any dietary preferences.

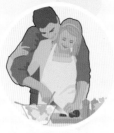

Cook together to get things sizzling.

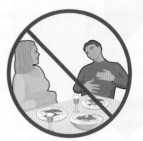

Keep portions small.

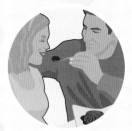

Don't forget dessert!

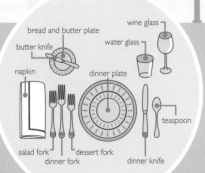

bread and butter plate

butter knife

napkin

wine glass

water glass

dinner plate

teaspoon

salad fork

dinner fork

dessert fork

dinner knife

Set a formal table to serve suggestive, aphrodisiac foods. You'll be all ready to follow up a proper dinner with some very improper conduct.

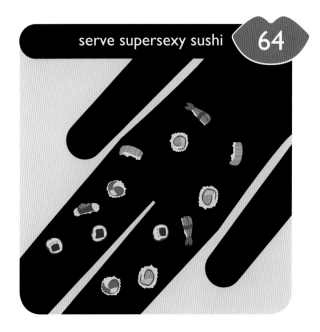

serve supersexy sushi **64**

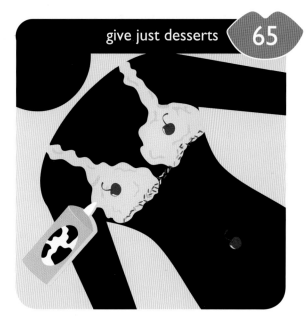

give just desserts **65**

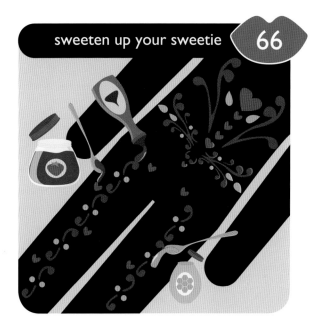

sweeten up your sweetie **66**

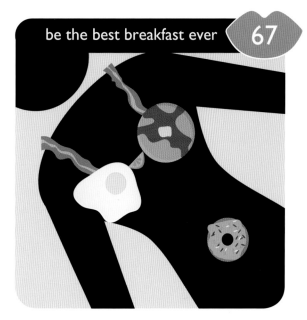

be the best breakfast ever **67**

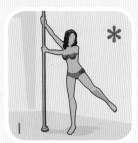

1 Reach up high on pole.

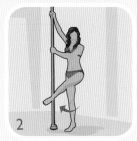

2 Swing leg for momentum.

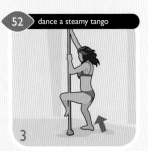

52 dance a steamy tango

3 Hook knee; push off ground.

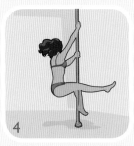

4 Extend leg to slow down.

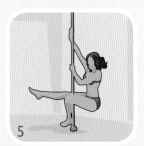

5 Spin as low as you dare.

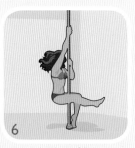

6 Land gracefully.

Pole dancing can boost confidence and tone muscles—with or without an audience. If you've got an inner showgirl (or showboy) to let out, order a pole for your home, or check out a pole-dancing exercise class at the gym.

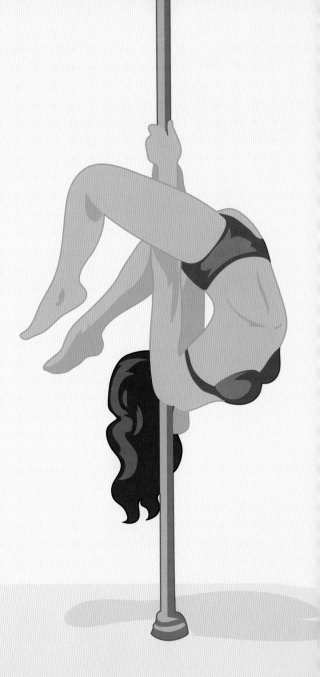

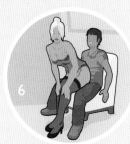

Slide back to standing.

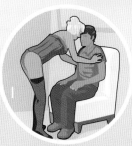

Lean in, greet your lover.

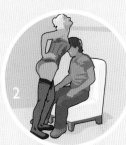

Let him enjoy the view.

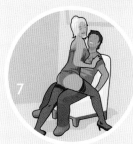

Turn forward, snuggle up.

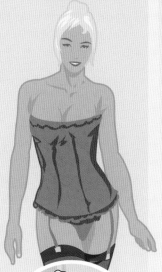

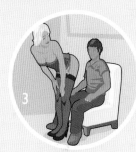

Turn around, bend over.

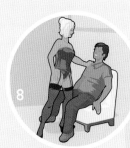

Move legs inside;
continue grinding.

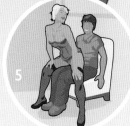

Straddle; rub up against him.

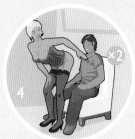

×2

Give yourself a
playful smack.

Some ladies like to sport a conceptual art piece downtown, while others rely on a trim and a little shaping to feel neat and tidy. Try these styles next time you need a new 'do.

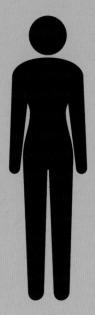

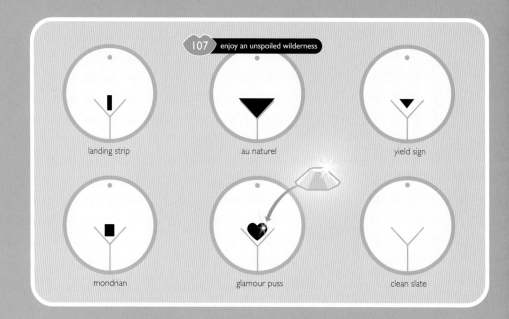

107 enjoy an unspoiled wilderness

landing strip

au naturel

yield sign

mondrian

glamour puss

clean slate

72   wax it all off

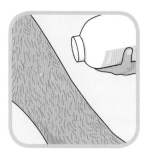

Apply talcum powder.

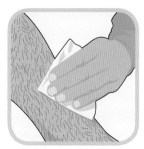

Rub powder into skin.

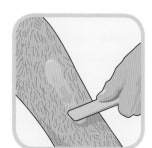

Add wax along hair growth.

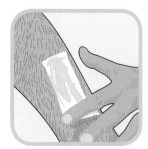

Smooth on cloth strip.

Most men get by with a simple pruning every now and then, but more aesthetically minded fellows will brave hot wax for an innovative look.

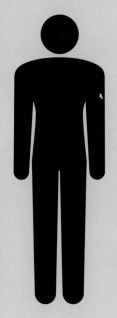

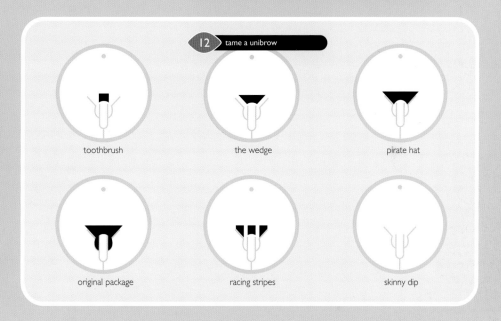

12 tame a unibrow

toothbrush

the wedge

pirate hat

original package

racing stripes

skinny dip

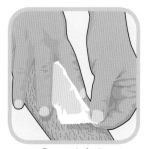

Grasp end of strip.

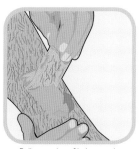

Pull opposite of hair growth.

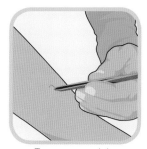

Tweeze any stray hairs.

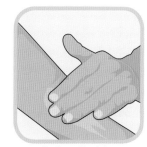

Apply soothing balm.

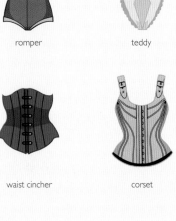

romper

teddy

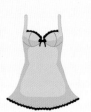

babydoll

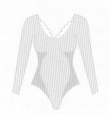

bodysuit

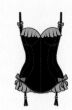

merry widow

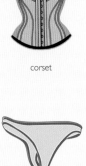

waist cincher

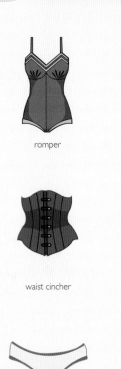

corset

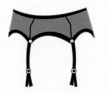

bustier

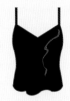

garter belt

camisole

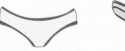

bikini panties

thong

g-string

boy shorts

rhumba panties

crotchless pantyhose

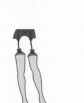

stockings

thigh-highs

catsuit

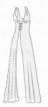

negligee

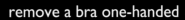

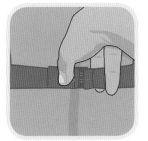
Insert index finger.

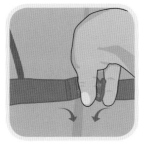
Gather the fabric.

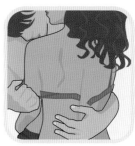
Pinch; release hooks slowly.

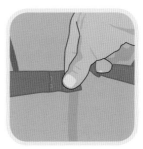
Slide strap off arm.

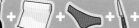

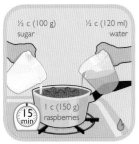
½ c (100 g) sugar
½ c (120 ml) water
15 min
1 c (150 g) raspberries
Cover pot and simmer.

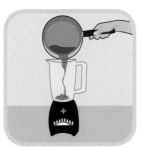
Blend.

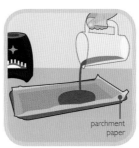
parchment paper
Pour onto lined baking pan.

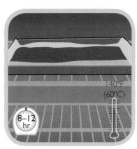
140°F (60°C)
8–12 hr.
Bake.

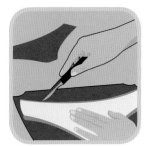
Use panties as a template.

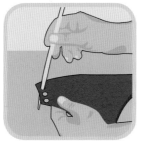
Poke holes with a chopstick.

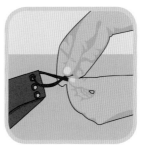
Tie together with licorice.

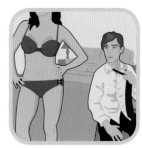
Serve at once!

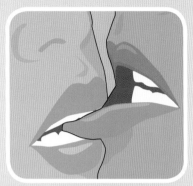

Gently bite lips.

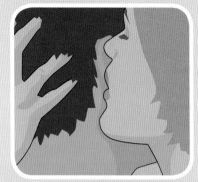

Massage scalp.

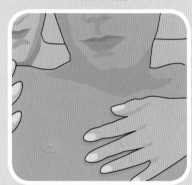

Nibble earlobes.

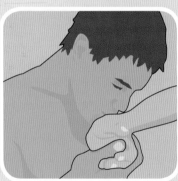

Kiss inside of wrists.

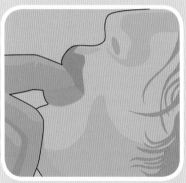

Suck on fingers.

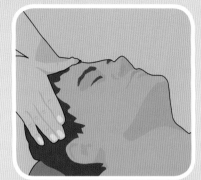

Caress chest.

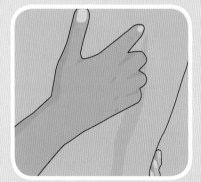

Lightly scratch back.

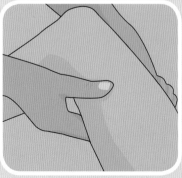

Tickle back of legs.

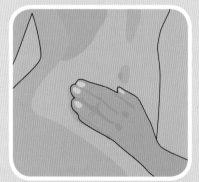

Stroke curve of hip bone.

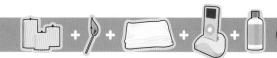 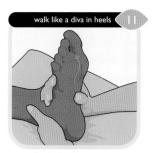 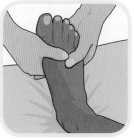 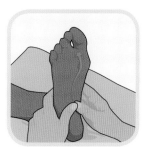 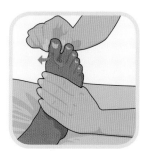

give a relaxing foot rub 77

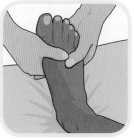
Stroke top of foot.

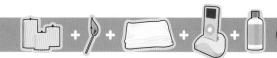
walk like a diva in heels 11
Apply circular pressure.

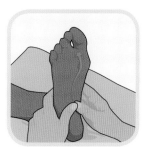
Glide up the central groove.

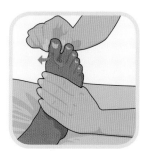
Rub and wiggle each toe.

entice with erotic massage 78

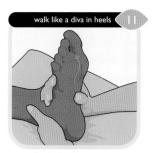
Set the romantic scene.

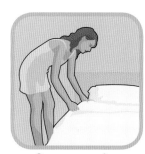
Cover massage surface.

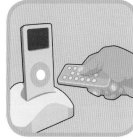
Put on some mood music.

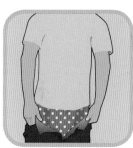
Have him strip down.

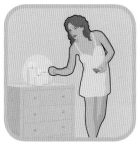
Create an erotic connection.

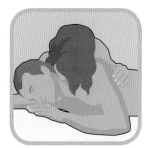
Warm massage oil in hands.

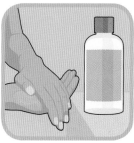
Massage sensually.

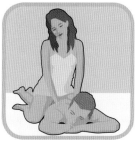
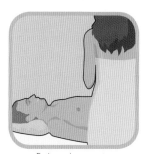
End on a happy note.

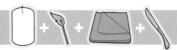

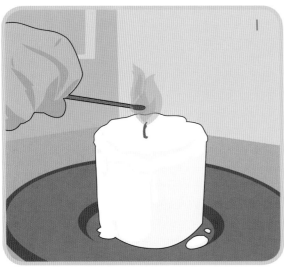

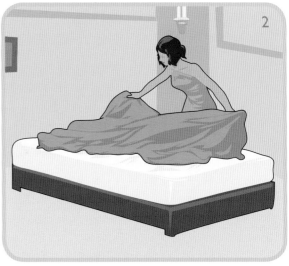

Light candle. (Pale-colored wax won't get as hot.)

Protect bedding with an old sheet.

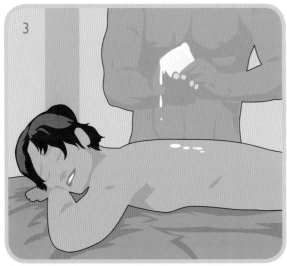

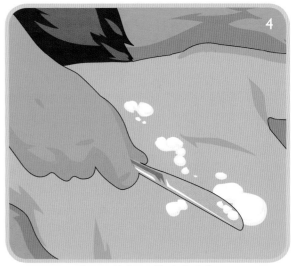

For cooler sensations, hold candle higher and drip wax.

Remove dried wax with a butter knife.

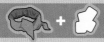

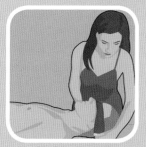
Blindfold your lover.

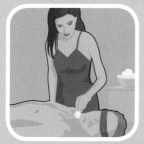
Introduce a novel sensation.

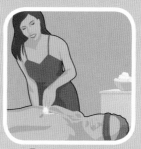
Trace item over body.

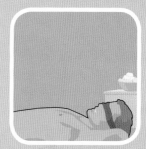
Tease sensitive spots.

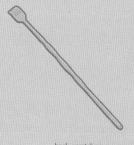
back-scratcher

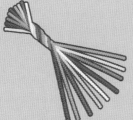
pipe cleaners

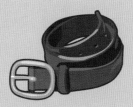
leather belt

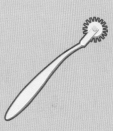
pinwheel

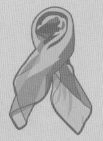
silk scarf

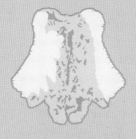
fur

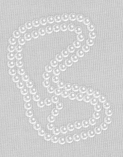
pearl necklace

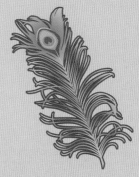
feather

Sex toys that target the g-spot come in a variety of shapes, and always have a bend or curve.

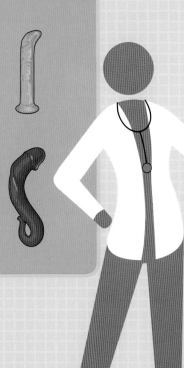

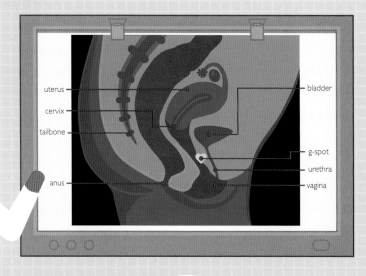

uterus — bladder

cervix

tailbone — g-spot

— urethra

anus — vagina

The g-spot is named for Dr. Ernst Gräfenberg, who first described it in 1950. To stimulate this sensitive tissue, insert curved fingers and press gently until you find a spot that feels a bit firmer.

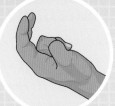

Let your fingers do the pleasing—after you've prepped properly.

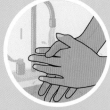

Wash hands well.

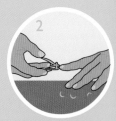

Clip nails short.

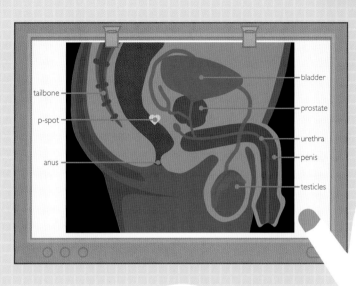

- tailbone
- p-spot
- anus
- bladder
- prostate
- urethra
- penis
- testicles

Prostate toys are specially designed to work the p-spot—and to stay put during sex.

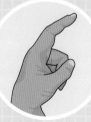

To stimulate the prostate (a.k.a., p-spot), insert one finger, feeling for a spot that is slightly raised. Press or rub gently, whichever your partner prefers.

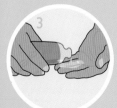

Pour a little lube.

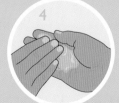

Rub hands to warm.

83 practice putting on a condom

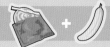 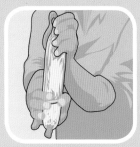

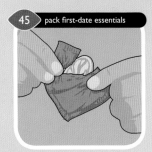

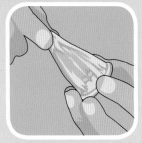

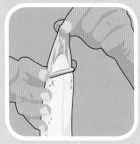

45 pack first-date essentials

Open package carefully.

Check that it's right side out.

Pinch the reservoir tip.

Roll down, pinching tip.

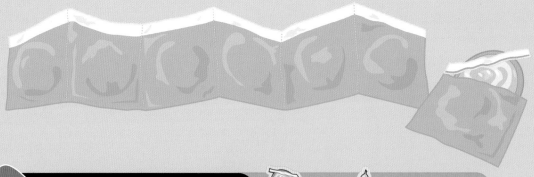

84 roll on a rubber hands-free

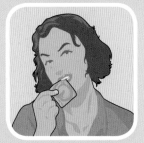

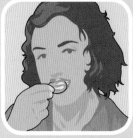

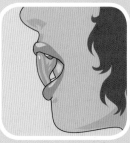

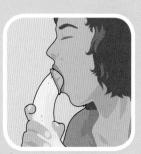

Remove from package.

Inhale slightly to inflate.

Hold tip with tongue.

Roll down using lips.

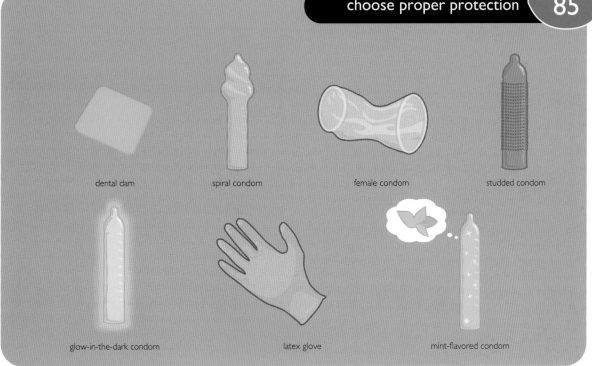

dental dam

spiral condom

female condom

studded condom

glow-in-the-dark condom

latex glove

mint-flavored condom

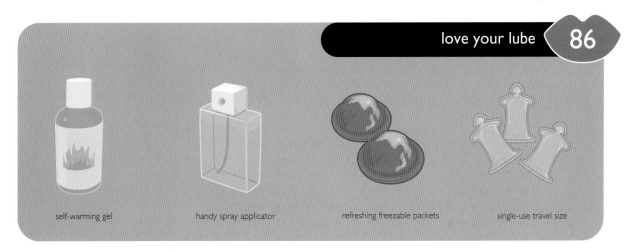

self-warming gel

handy spray applicator

refreshing freezable packets

single-use travel size

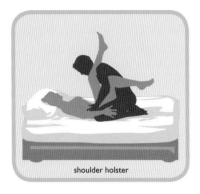
shoulder holster

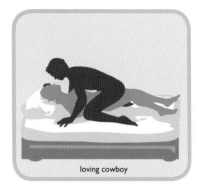
loving cowboy

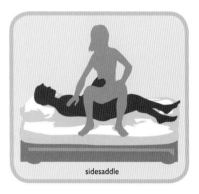
sidesaddle

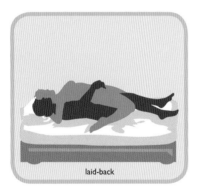
laid-back

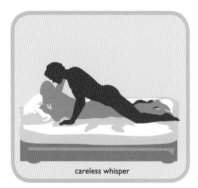
careless whisper

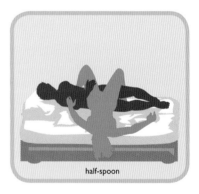
half-spoon

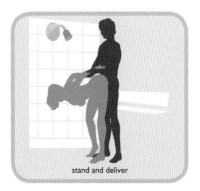
stand and deliver

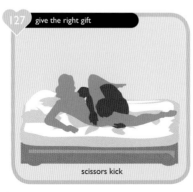

127 give the right gift

scissors kick

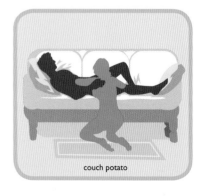
couch potato

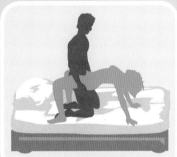

bridge to somewhere

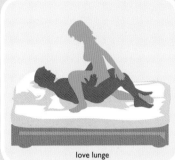

love lunge

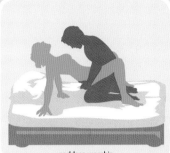

goddess worship

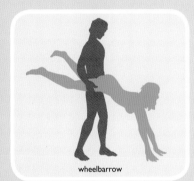

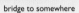

wheelbarrow

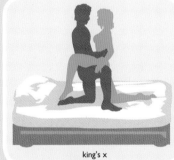

king's x

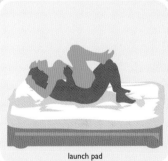

launch pad

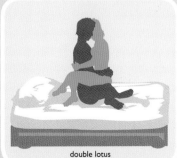

double lotus

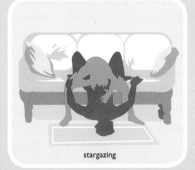

stargazing

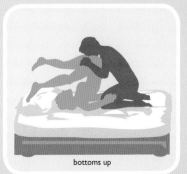

bottoms up

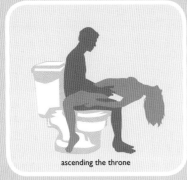

ascending the throne

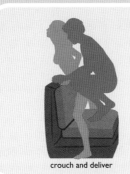

crouch and deliver

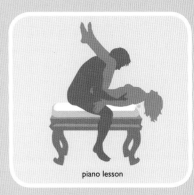

piano lesson

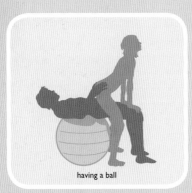

having a ball

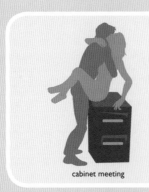

cabinet meeting

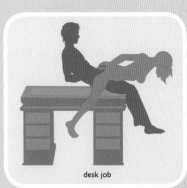

desk job

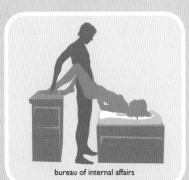

bureau of internal affairs

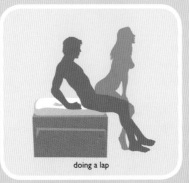

doing a lap

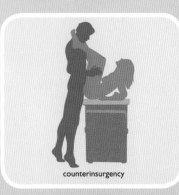

counterinsurgency

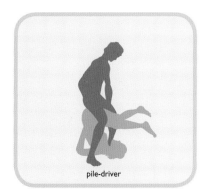

pile-driver

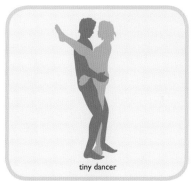

tiny dancer

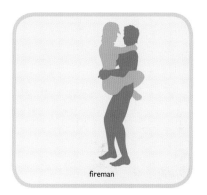

fireman

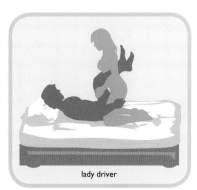

lady driver

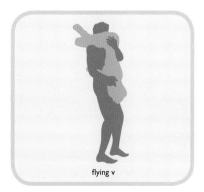

flying v

bond with couples' yoga 123

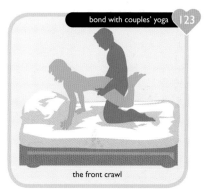

the front crawl

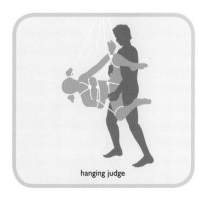

hanging judge

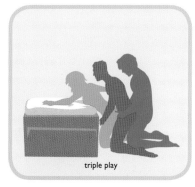

triple play

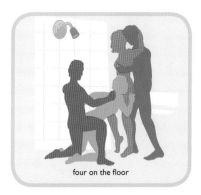

four on the floor

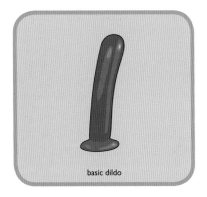

basic dildo

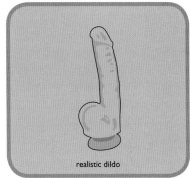

realistic dildo

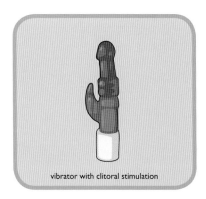

vibrator with clitoral stimulation

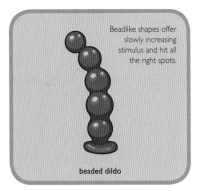

Beadlike shapes offer slowly increasing stimulus and hit all the right spots.

beaded dildo

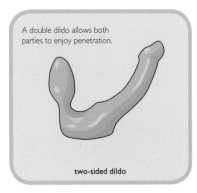

butt plug

82 pleasure the p-spot

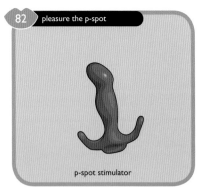

p-spot stimulator

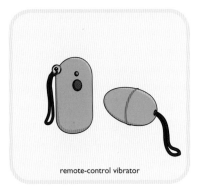

remote-control vibrator

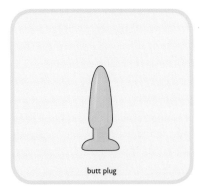

A double dildo allows both parties to enjoy penetration.

two-sided dildo

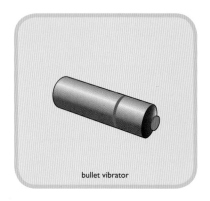

bullet vibrator

A stretchy ring grips him tight while soft nubs rub her the right way.

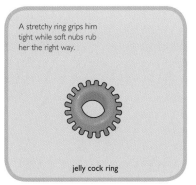

jelly cock ring

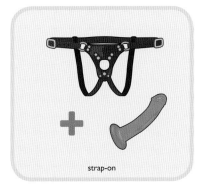

strap-on

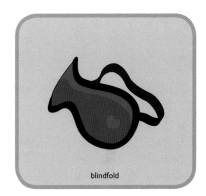

blindfold

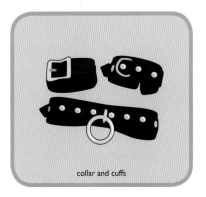

collar and cuffs

They may look painful, but nipple clamps can be adjusted to deliver just a tantalizing squeeze.

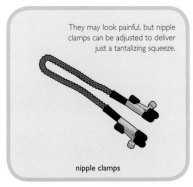

nipple clamps

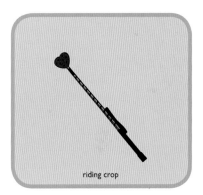

riding crop

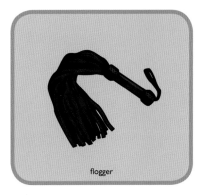

flogger

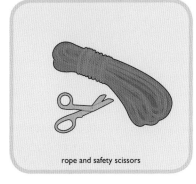

rope and safety scissors

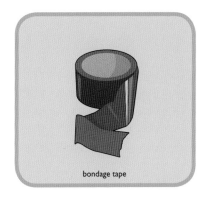

bondage tape

Talk about your naughtiest (or silliest) fantasies and agree to dress up for each other. Try role-playing a scene in which, for example, a dusty cowboy hires a saucy French maid to clean up for him—and things get very dirty in the process!

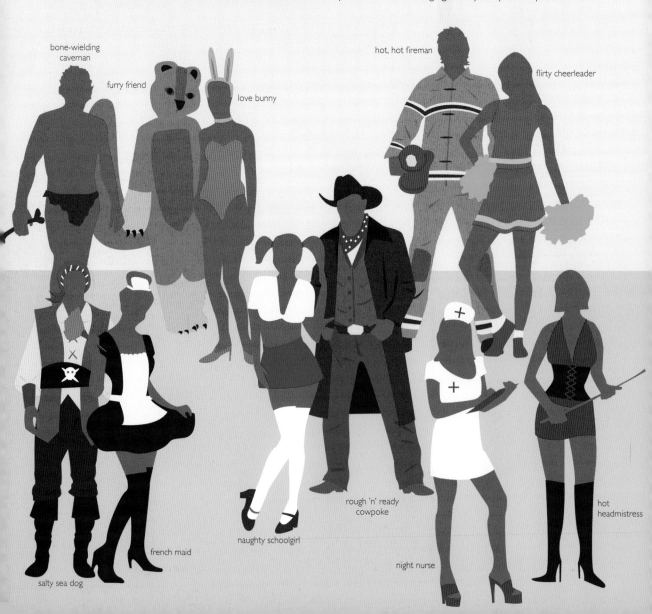

bone-wielding caveman

furry friend

love bunny

hot, hot fireman

flirty cheerleader

salty sea dog

french maid

naughty schoolgirl

rough 'n' ready cowpoke

night nurse

hot headmistress

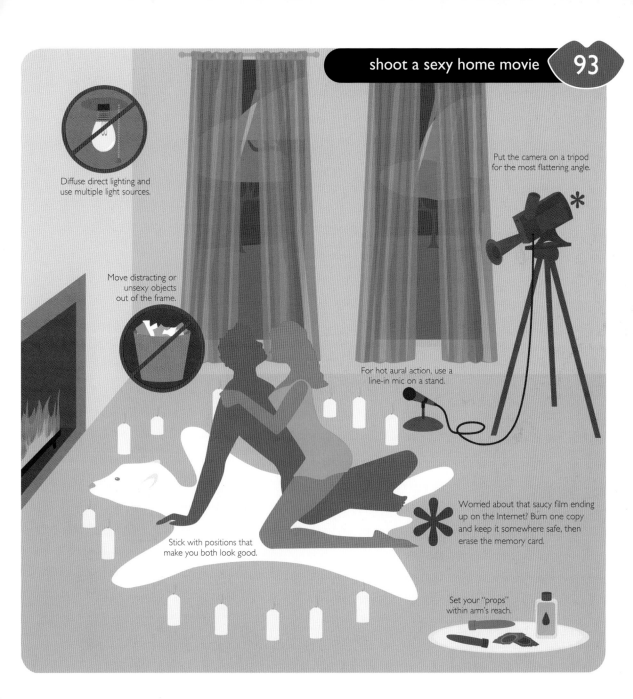

Diffuse direct lighting and use multiple light sources.

Put the camera on a tripod for the most flattering angle.

Move distracting or unsexy objects out of the frame.

For hot aural action, use a line-in mic on a stand.

Worried about that saucy film ending up on the Internet? Burn one copy and keep it somewhere safe, then erase the memory card.

Stick with positions that make you both look good.

Set your "props" within arm's reach.

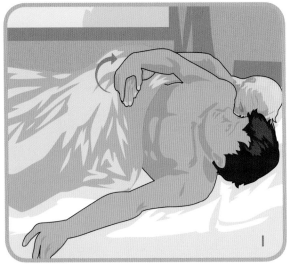

Gently extract yourself.

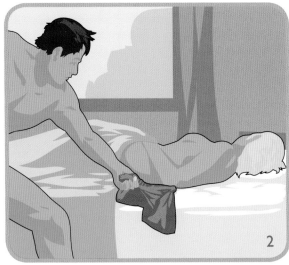

Quietly locate all your belongings.

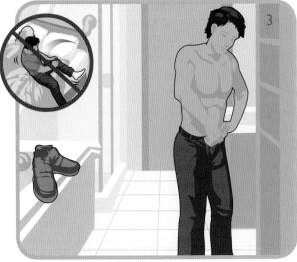

Exit the bedroom to dress.

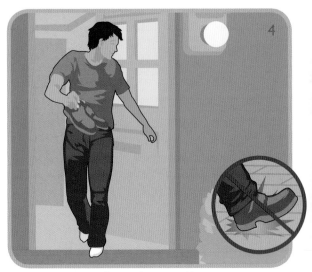

Put your shoes on outside.

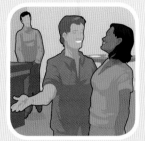

Focus on your new partner.

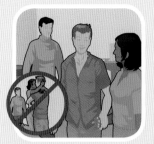

Be affectionate.

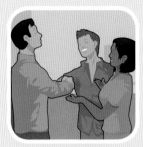

Make introductions.

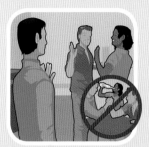

Move on politely.

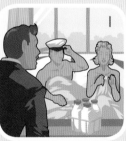

Cover up quickly.

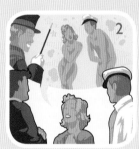

Offer an explanation.

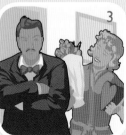

Apologize profusely.

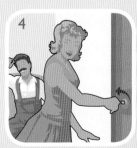

Next time, be prepared.

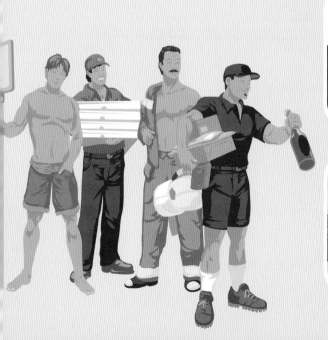

For sexy restraints at a moment's notice (without raising the eyebrows of your guests), rig up this clever bondage bed. The loose ends can be hidden under the bed skirt.

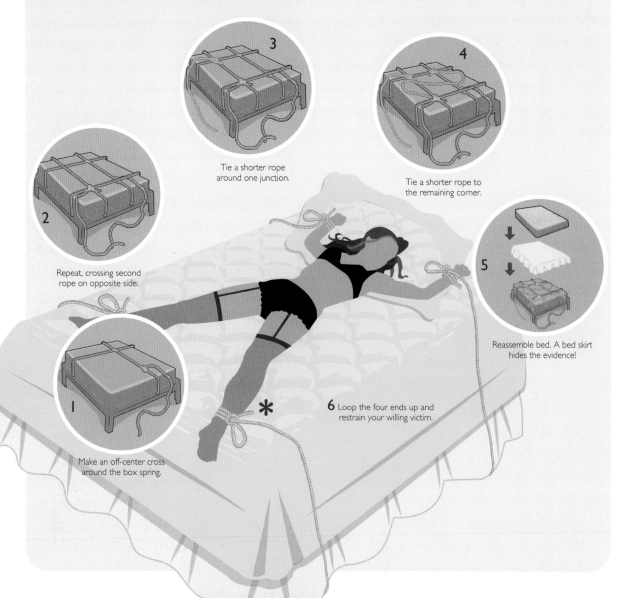

Tie a shorter rope around one junction.

Tie a shorter rope to the remaining corner.

Repeat, crossing second rope on opposite side.

Reassemble bed. A bed skirt hides the evidence!

Make an off-center cross around the box spring.

6 Loop the four ends up and restrain your willing victim.

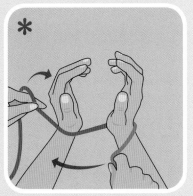

Create a figure eight.

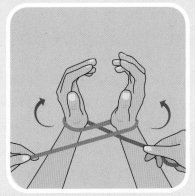

Repeat.

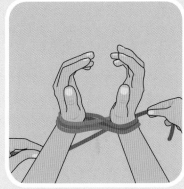

Repeat again for extra security.

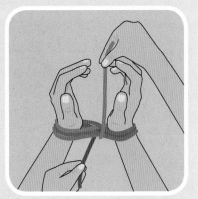

Wrap the ends.

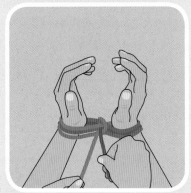

Tie off in the center.

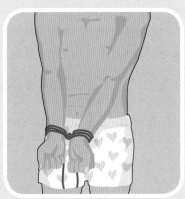

Enjoy the sexy struggle.

When experimenting with any edgy activity, be sure to agree on safe words beforehand. Safe words let you playfully beg "stop!" when you really mean "don't stop," while assuring that your partner really will stop on "red" when you've had enough.

Say "green" when you mean "This is great! More please!"

Say "yellow" when you mean "I like that, but please slow down a little."

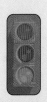

Say "red" when you mean "Stop right now. I'm not having fun anymore."

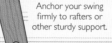

Anchor your swing firmly to rafters or other sturdy support.

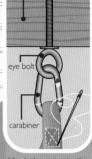

plank

eye bolt

carabiner

Hook the swing to the plank with a carabiner so you can easily take it down when you're done swingin'.

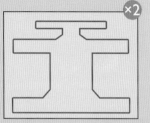

×2

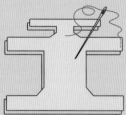

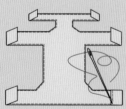

Cut out pattern from heavy canvas or leather. Sew securely.

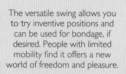

The versatile swing allows you to try inventive positions and can be used for bondage, if desired. People with limited mobility find it offers a new world of freedom and pleasure.

Strengthen seams with rivets.

Add a pillow for style and comfort.

Heavy nylon straps are strong enough to support your swing. For that classic bondage look, opt for metal chains instead.

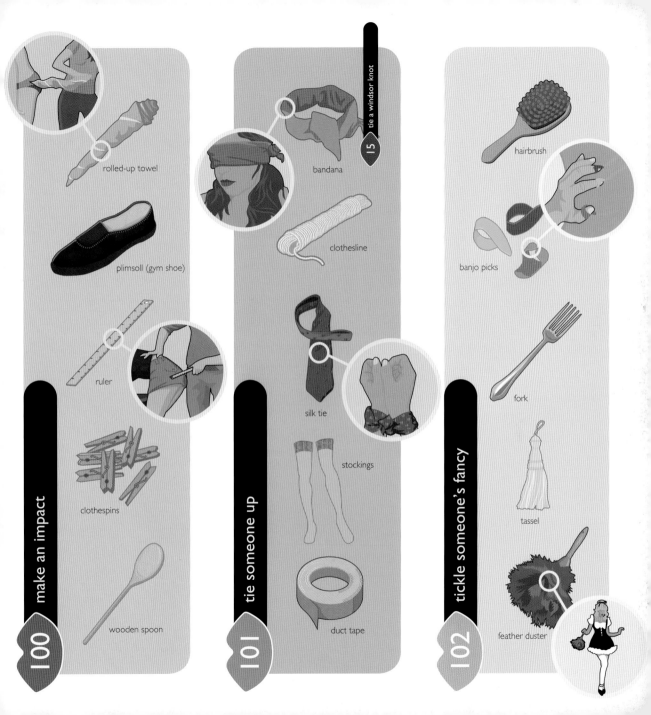

rolled-up towel

plimsoll (gym shoe)

ruler

clothespins

wooden spoon

100 make an impact

15 tie a windsor knot

bandana

clothesline

silk tie

stockings

duct tape

101 tie someone up

hairbrush

banjo picks

fork

tassel

feather duster

102 tickle someone's fancy

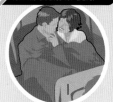

fold his clothes for travel

Get things started
under a blanket.

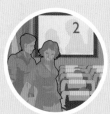

Wait until fellow travelers
are distracted . . .

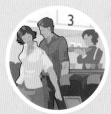

. . . or go when the aisle
is blocked for others.

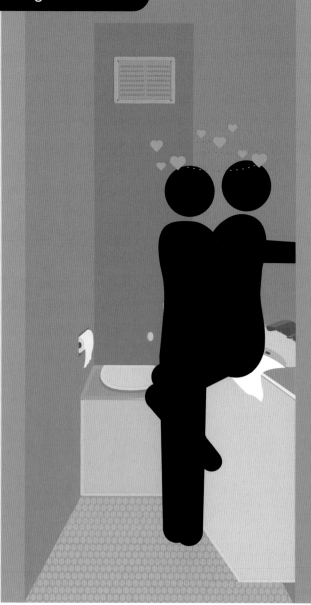

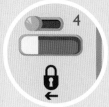

Be sure the door is locked.

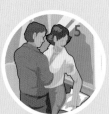

Put down paper towels.

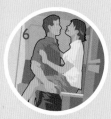

A skirt makes
undressing unnecessary.

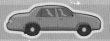

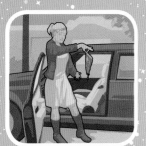

Be sure car is clean.

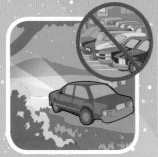

Park in a secluded spot.

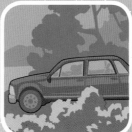

Turn off all lights.

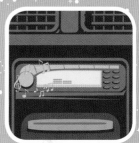

Turn radio down low.

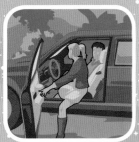

Move to the passenger seat.

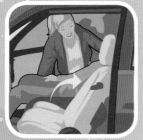

Recline the seat slightly.

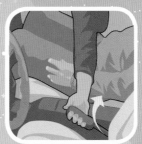

Apply the parking brake.

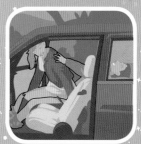

Time to park 'n' ride.

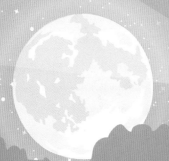

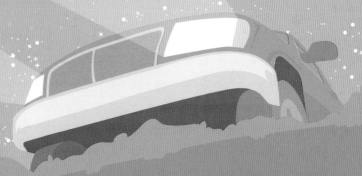

 Unless you're planning a very long ride, it's okay to play the radio—most car batteries last for four to eight hours. If you know that your battery is weak, don't risk getting stranded.

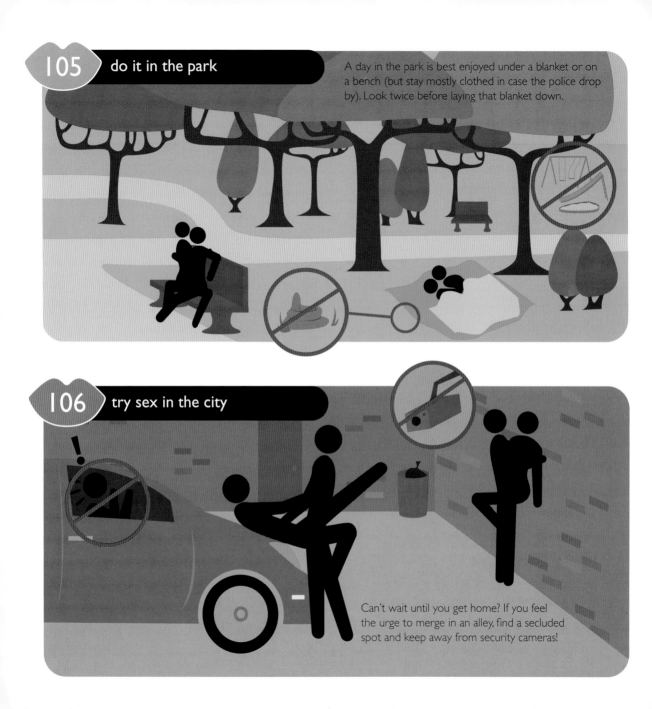

105 do it in the park

A day in the park is best enjoyed under a blanket or on a bench (but stay mostly clothed in case the police drop by). Look twice before laying that blanket down.

106 try sex in the city

Can't wait until you get home? If you feel the urge to merge in an alley, find a secluded spot and keep away from security cameras!

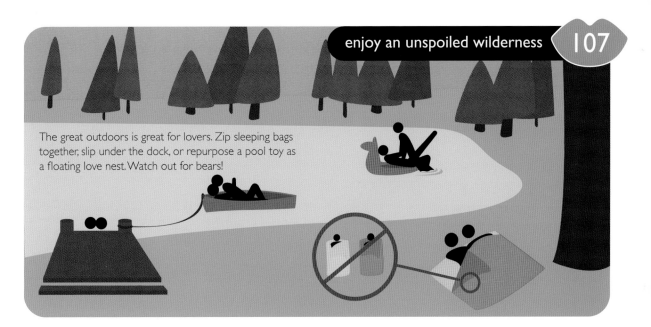

The great outdoors is great for lovers. Zip sleeping bags together, slip under the dock, or repurpose a pool toy as a floating love nest. Watch out for bears!

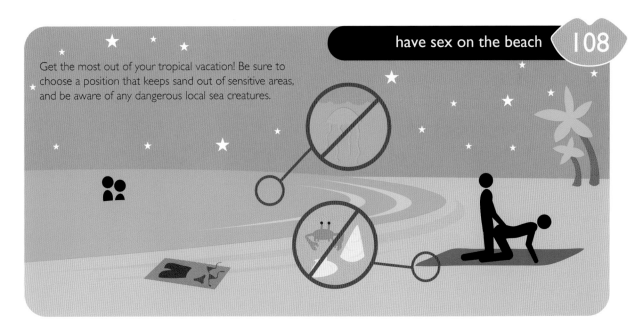

Get the most out of your tropical vacation! Be sure to choose a position that keeps sand out of sensitive areas, and be aware of any dangerous local sea creatures.

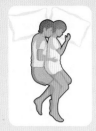

loving relationship

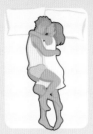

hot and exciting

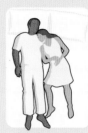

nurturing partner

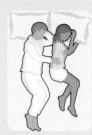

trusting relationship

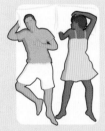

after a fight

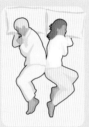

tired but loving

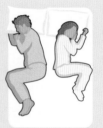

tension in relationship

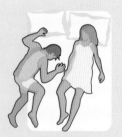

wants to escape

110 spoon comfortably

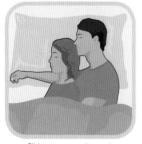

Slide arm up under neck.

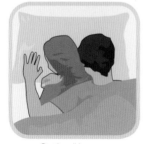

Gently roll her over.

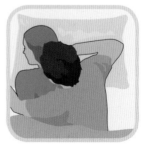

Free trapped arm.

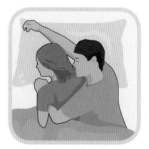

Extend arm above her.

Ask your dreamboat to tell you about his or her dreamlife, then compare the elements to these time-tested interpretations for a sneak peak into your sweetie's psyche.

ring
commitment

whip
domination, obedience

coat
secrecy or protection

dragon
powerful urges

wolf
ravenous desires, unfulfilled appetites

bull
forceful masculinity

rose
female genitalia, menstruation, love

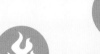
fire
passion or envy

fountain
romantic energy, orgasm

key into lock
the sexual act

rocket
phallus, soaring to new heights

snake
mystical sexual energy

orchid
sexuality, sensuality

moon
woman, secret, cyclical

broken object
possible breakup

heart
emotional life, feelings

candle
phallus or illumination

sword
phallus, truth, power

cup
feminity, love, truth

gloves
female genitalia, womb, protection

fence
separation or obstacle

net
good catch or feeling trapped

game
playing games with your lover

cork popping
ejaculation

mermaid
enticing, virginal, dangerous

boot
dominant female sexuality

hotel
impersonal, impermanent

bond

have a sweet morning after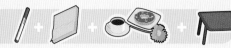

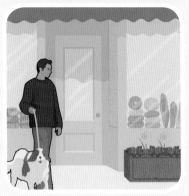
Do your research in advance.

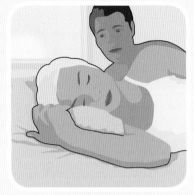
Sneak out of bed.

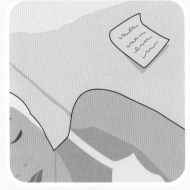
Leave a "be right back" note.

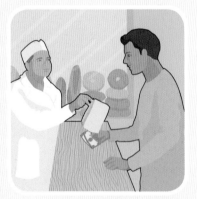
Get the goodies.

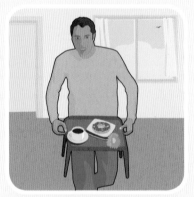
Set up your feast.

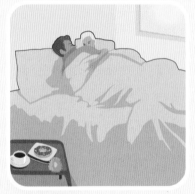
Time to rise and shine!

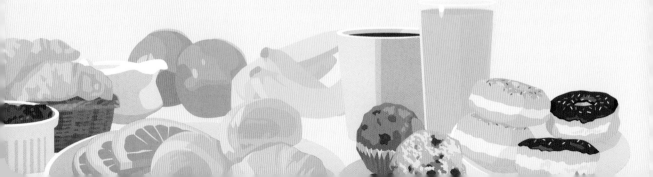

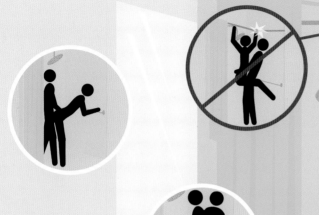

There's room for everyone under an extra-wide shower head.

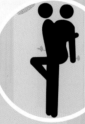

Aim that spray right where you want it with a handheld shower nozzle.

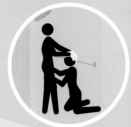

There's nothing hot about a concussion—put down a bath mat when trysting in the tub!

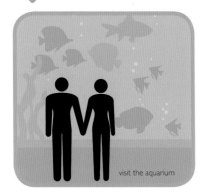

visit the aquarium

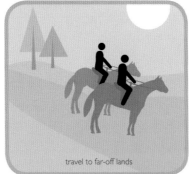

travel to far-off lands

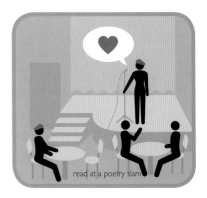

read at a poetry slam

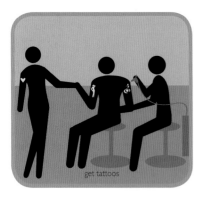

get tattoos

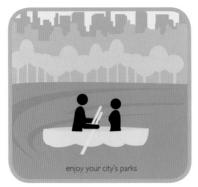

enjoy your city's parks

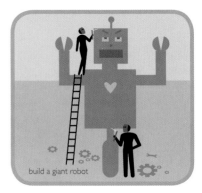

build a giant robot

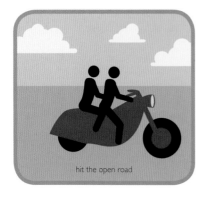

hit the open road

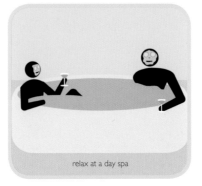

relax at a day spa

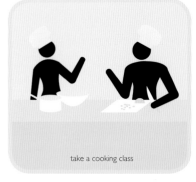

take a cooking class

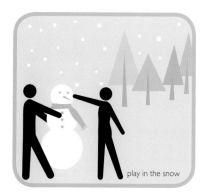

play in the snow

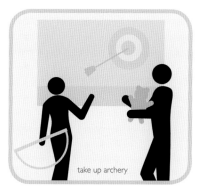

take up archery

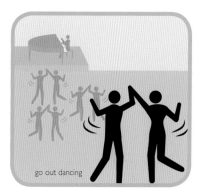

go out dancing

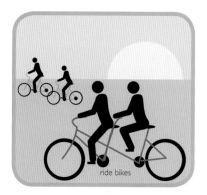

ride bikes

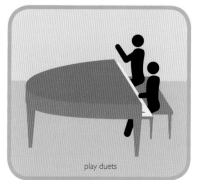

play duets

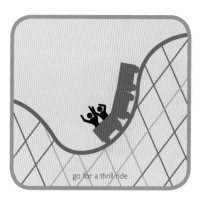

go for a thrill ride

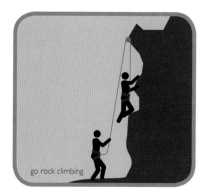

go rock climbing

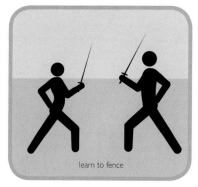

learn to fence

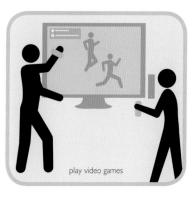

play video games

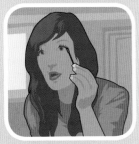
Look your best.

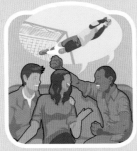
Find your common interests.

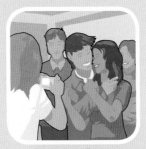
Display your affection.

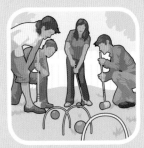
Participate in their activities.

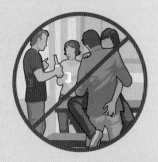

Your honey's friends want to see that you two are in love—but they don't need to see it in graphic detail. Be courteous and go easy on the PDA.

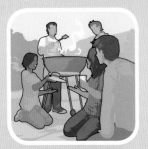
Pick a low-key event.

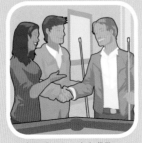
Introduce people he'll like.

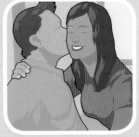
Pay him plenty of attention.

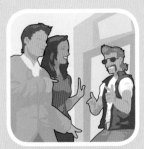
Save him from weirdos.

Meeting Mom and Dad for the first time can be scary. Luckily there are a few basic things every parent dreams of seeing when their child brings home a special someone.

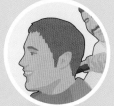

Clean yourself up.

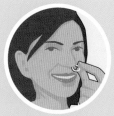

Remove piercings.

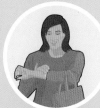

Be on time.

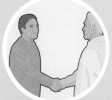

Act confident and friendly.

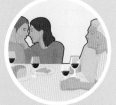

Show that you're smitten.

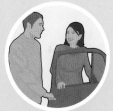

Be a gentleman.

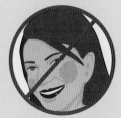

Don't look like a trollop.

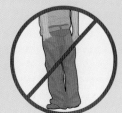

Don't dress like a teen.

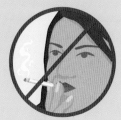

Don't smoke!

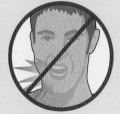

Don't be a boor.

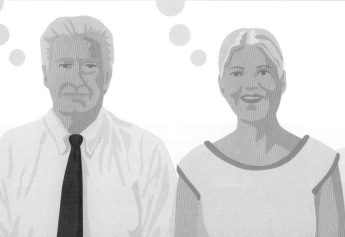

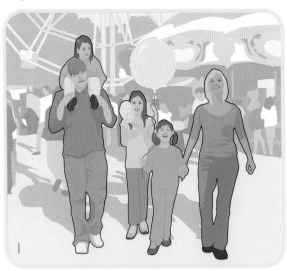

Arrange a kid-friendly date.

39 score at a kid's soccer game

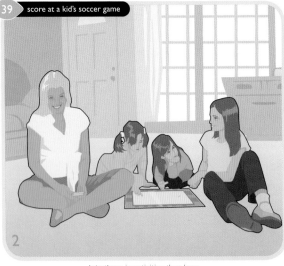

Join them in activities they love.

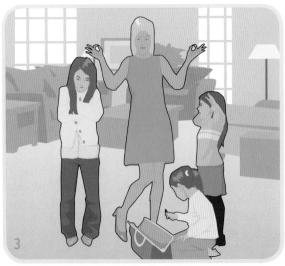

Remain calm when they misbehave.

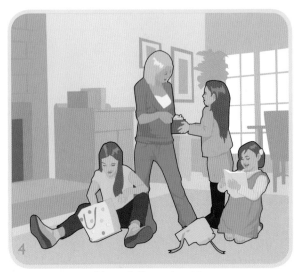

Bring small gifts once in a while.

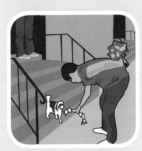

Bring a gift.

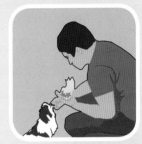

Always carry treats.

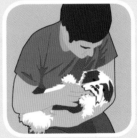

Show some love.

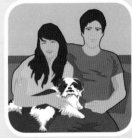

Be inclusive when at home.

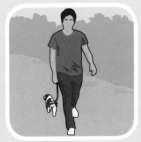

Be the alpha dog.

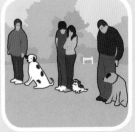

Join in at obedience class.

❤ 120 have a healthy fight

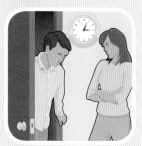

Only fight when it's worth it.

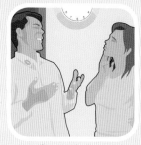

Give him a chance.

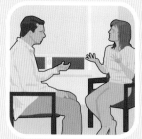

Sit down to discuss.

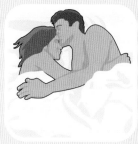

Don't go to bed angry.

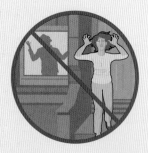

A healthy fight is all about listening to each other respectfully. Throwing china and accusations, or storming out of the house, may be satisfying for a moment, but the drama won't lead to long-term stability and trust.

❤ 121 channel your aggressions

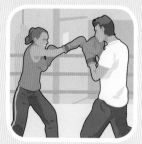

Take boxing class together.

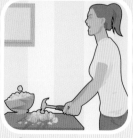

Break unimportant objects.

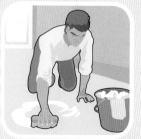

Scrub away your anger.

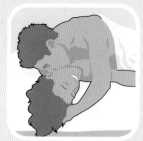

Work it all out in bed.

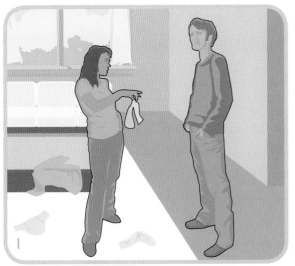

Listen to your partner's concerns.

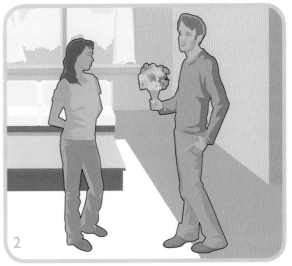

Bring home a small gift.

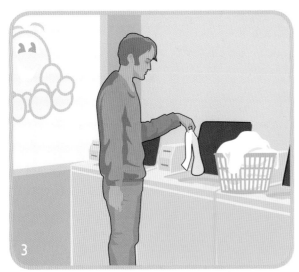

Make it clear that your behavior has changed.

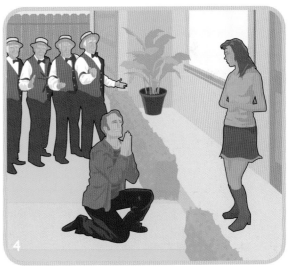

Get creative.

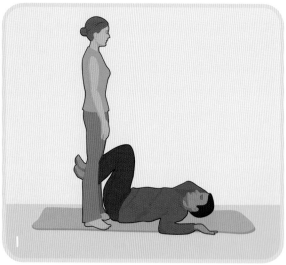

1

Lie on back with legs bent between partner's legs.

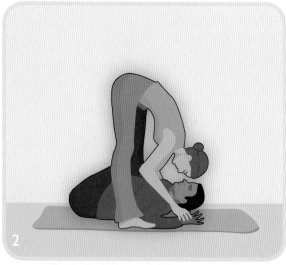

2

Place feet just inside partner's hipbones; touch hands.

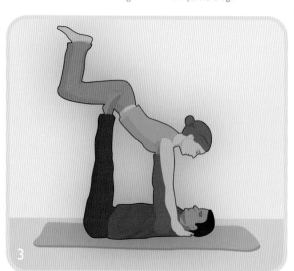

3

Straighten legs to lift partner; support her shoulders.

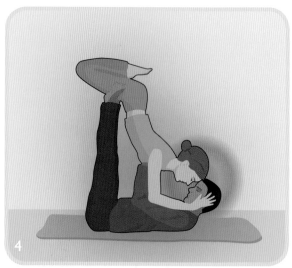

4

Partner bends knees, brings hands to your face.

Chakras are points that control energy flow to areas of the body. To take advantage of their cosmic power, sit back-to-back with your partner so that your chakras line up. (A pillow will help even out any height discrepancies.) Then concentrate together on each, starting at the bottom with the root chakra.

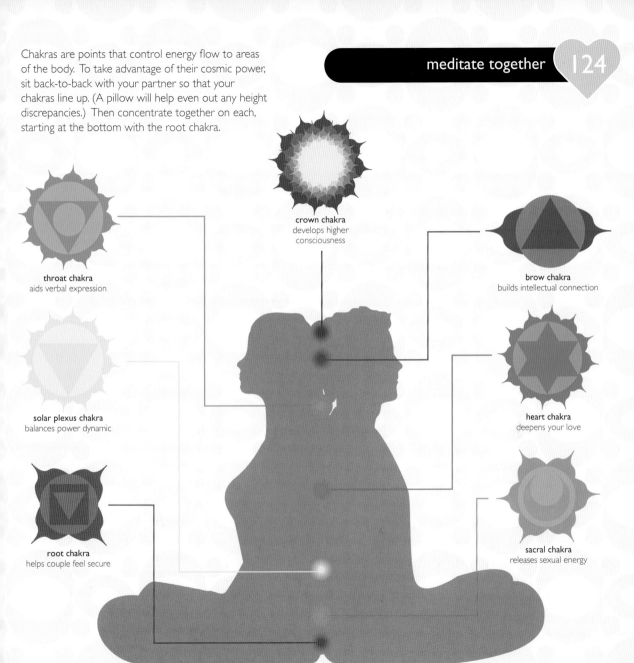

crown chakra
develops higher consciousness

throat chakra
aids verbal expression

brow chakra
builds intellectual connection

solar plexus chakra
balances power dynamic

heart chakra
deepens your love

root chakra
helps couple feel secure

sacral chakra
releases sexual energy

125 play the sexy stranger game

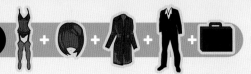

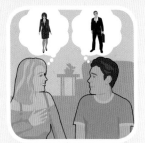

Agree on fantasy details.

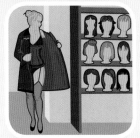

Dress the part.

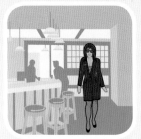

Arrive separately.

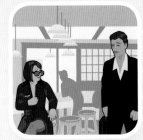

Flirt with your eyes.

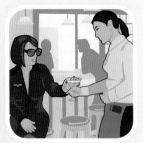

Send your lover a drink.

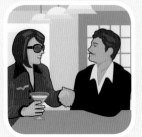

Introduce yourself.

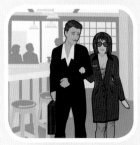

Complete the seduction.

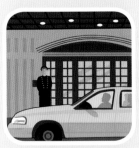

Spend the night at a hotel.

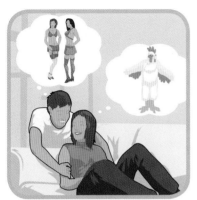

Agree on what you want; set boundaries.

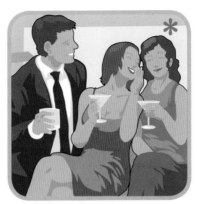

Approach an acquaintance.

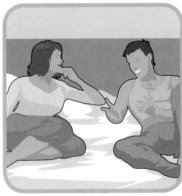

Relax together.

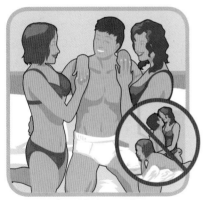

Spread the love equally.

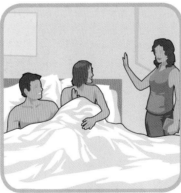

Say goodnight.

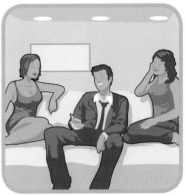

Discuss how it went.

The hardest part of setting up a threesome may be picking the right person. Both total strangers and close friends can be awkward choices. Try hitting it off with a casual acquaintance for maximum comfort with minimal risk.

127 give the right gift

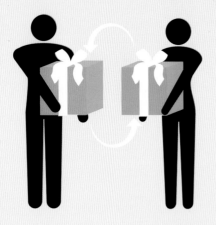

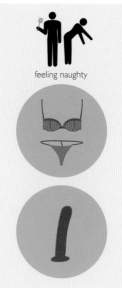

feeling naughty

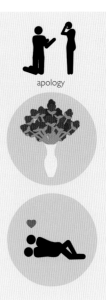

apology

128 leave a sneaky love note

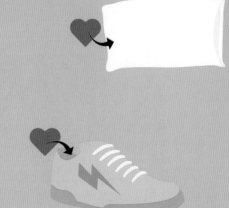

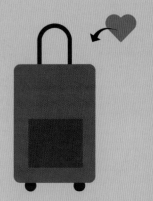

With love notes, it's really just the thought that counts. Write down one little thing that you love about your sweetie—or one little thing you'll want to do to her when she gets home!

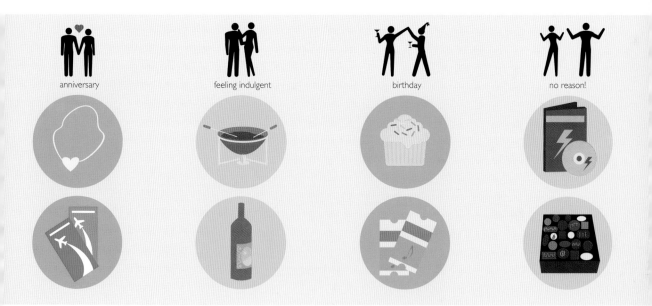

anniversary

feeling indulgent

birthday

no reason!

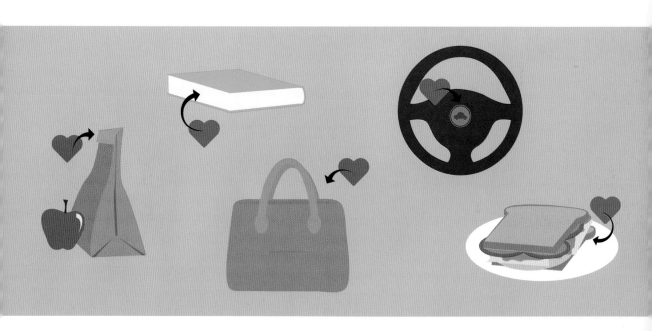

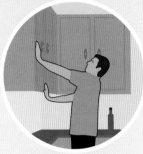

Close whatever you open.

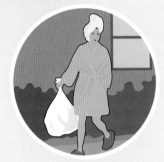

Take turns taking
out the trash.

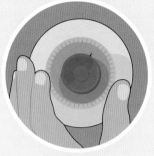

Don't power-trip on
the thermostat.

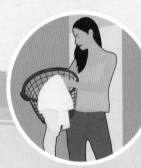

Put dirty clothes
in the hamper.

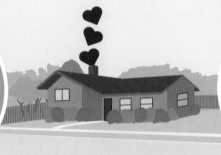

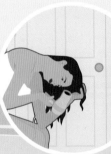

Shut the door
when blow-drying.

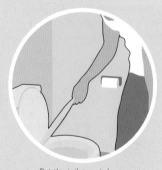

Put the toilet seat down.

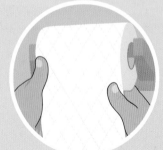

Replace the toilet paper.

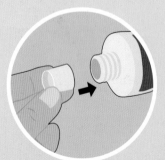

Put the cap back on
the toothpaste.

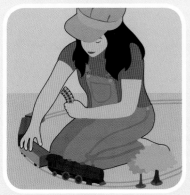
Keep up with your hobbies.

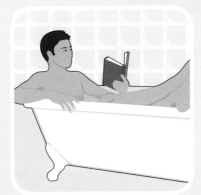
Savor alone time.

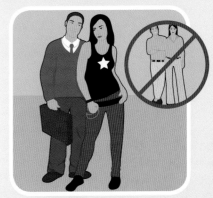
Maintain your personal style.

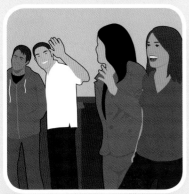
Make time for friends.

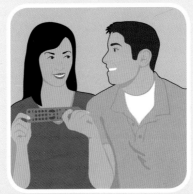
Assert your right to the remote.

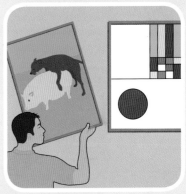
Mix and match your decor items.

You fell in love with each other's unique personalities. So don't lose your lovable, individualistic traits, and don't pressure your partner to become a clone. Vive la différence!

throw a crazy theme party

Entertaining as a couple doesn't have to mean the same old dinner party or movie night. Throw a party that reflects who you are—or who you wish you could be!

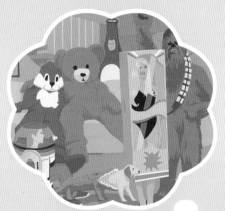

Host a costume party and let your friends show off their creativity.

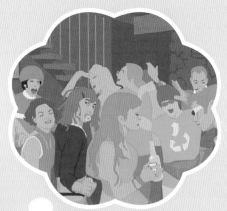

Do you miss the '90s? Have a crazy rave party and relive the madness.

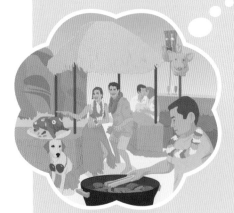

Throw a luau and get all your friends lei'd.

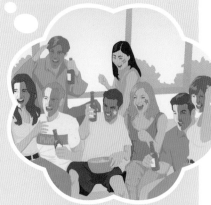

Celebrate the big game by inviting friendly rivals over for beer and snacks.

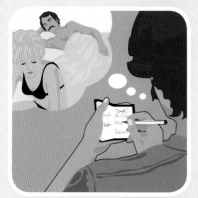

Invite your favorite sexy friends.

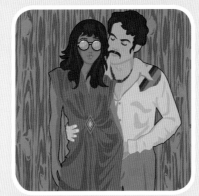

Instruct guests to dress in '70s finery.

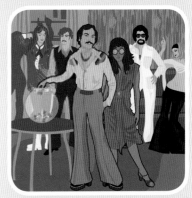

Arriving men drop their keys in a bowl.

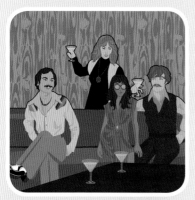

Encourage guests to meet and mingle.

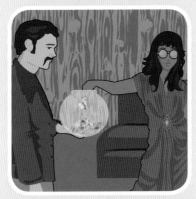

Later in the night, ladies pick a set of keys.

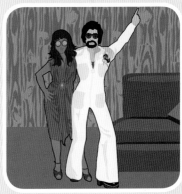

The lucky key owner is her date.

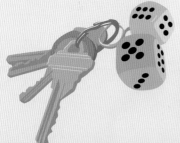

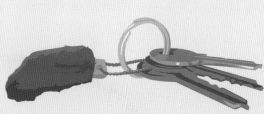

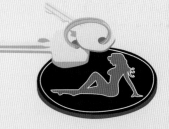

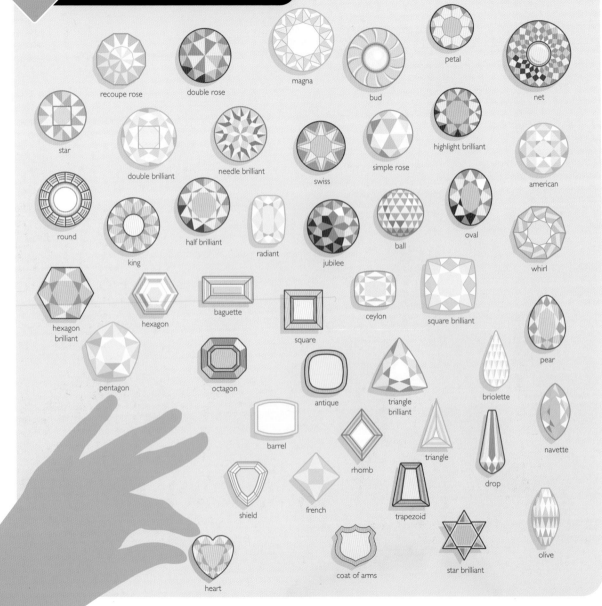

recoupe rose

double rose

magna

bud

petal

net

star

double brilliant

needle brilliant

swiss

simple rose

highlight brilliant

american

round

king

half brilliant

radiant

jubilee

ball

oval

whirl

hexagon brilliant

hexagon

baguette

ceylon

square brilliant

pear

pentagon

octagon

square

antique

triangle brilliant

briolette

navette

barrel

rhomb

triangle

drop

shield

french

trapezoid

olive

heart

coat of arms

star brilliant

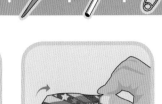

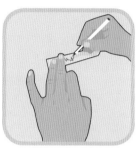

Snip from any paper source.

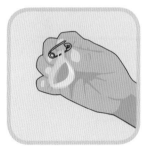

Fold in half lengthwise.

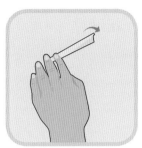

Fold in half again.

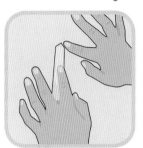

Fold the end into a point.

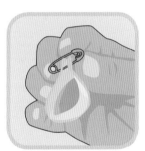

Write an inscription.

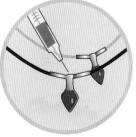

Make a loop.

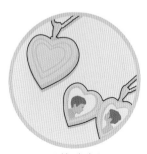

Secure with a safety pin.

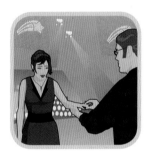

Ask for her hand.

explore ring alternatives **135**

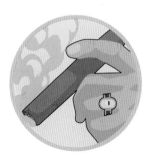

cigar band

vial of your blood

matching lockets

half-and-half tattoos

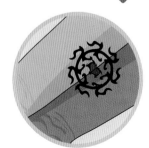

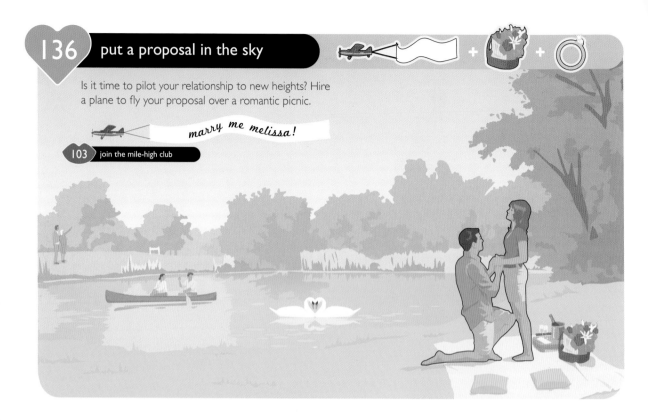

136 put a proposal in the sky

Is it time to pilot your relationship to new heights? Hire a plane to fly your proposal over a romantic picnic.

marry me melissa!

103 join the mile-high club

137 rock her world from jail

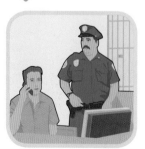

Call for help from jail.

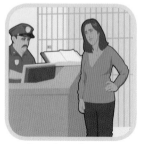

Say you're a prisoner . . .

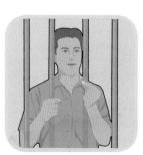

. . . of love.

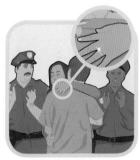

Give her the ring.

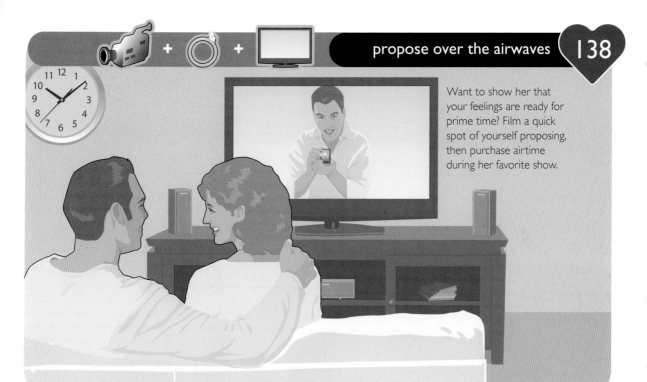

Want to show her that your feelings are ready for prime time? Film a quick spot of yourself proposing, then purchase airtime during her favorite show.

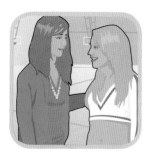

Enlist a cheerleader's help.

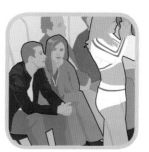

Sit courtside.

Ted marry Alice!

Enjoy the halftime show!

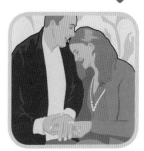

Give him the ring.

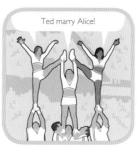

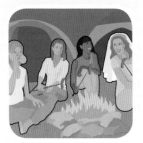

Party in the great outdoors.

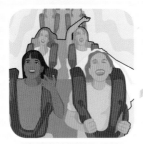

Thrill her at a theme park.

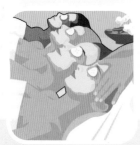

Relax at a day spa.

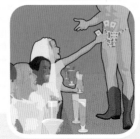

Get an eyeful at a strip club.

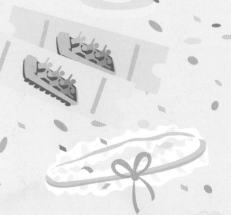

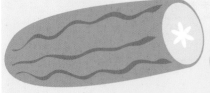

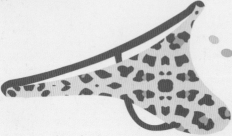

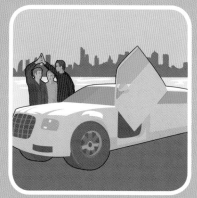

Provide safe transport.

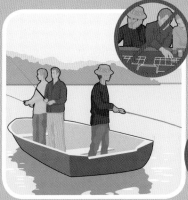

Pick an activity he likes.

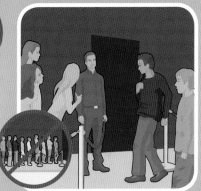

Book the venue in advance.

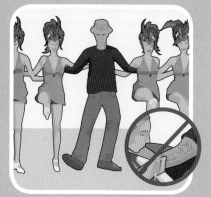

Keep behavior fairly sane.

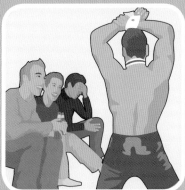

Plan a funny surprise.

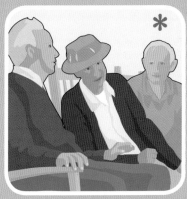

Keep the memories private.

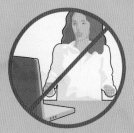

 If you plan a night he'll always remember, there should be no reason to store the pictures online. Your pal's wife-to-be and his future employers will appreciate your discretion.

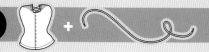

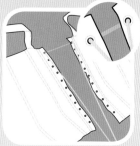
Lay it flat; lace the top holes.

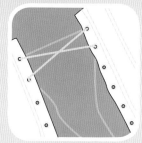
Cross; lace into next holes.

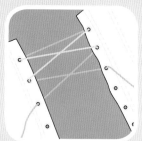
Cross beneath; lace out.

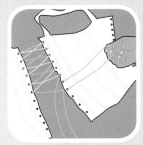
Stop midway; make a loop.

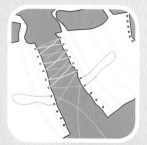
Make a facing loop.

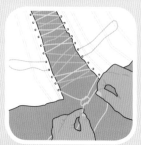
Lace to bottom; tie.

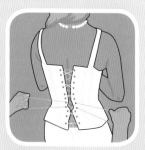
Put on; use loops to tighten.

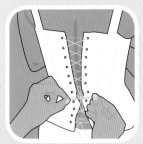
Tie the loops together.

143 toss the garter

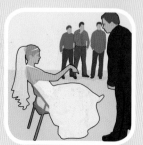
Come when beckoned.

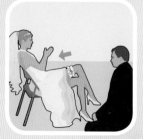
Slide bride's skirt up.

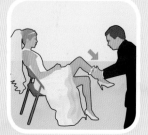
Remove garter.

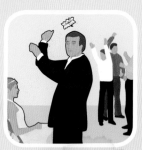
Toss to unmarried men.

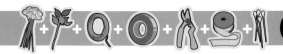
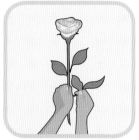

Remove leaves and thorns.

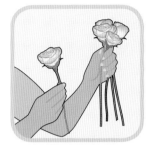

Group together.

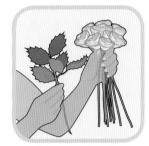

Add greenery beneath.

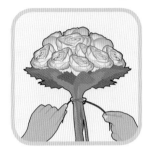

Secure with florist wire.

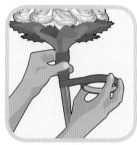

Wrap with florist tape.

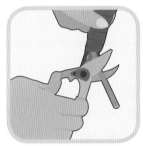

Trim the stems.

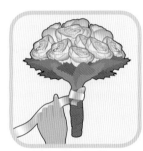

Adorn with satin ribbon.

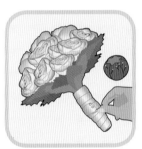

Fasten with pins.

make a boutonniere | 145

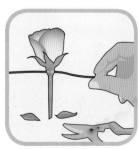

Trim rose; insert florist wire.

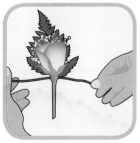

Add greens; wrap the wire.

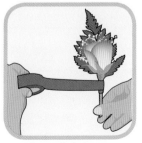

Cover with florist tape.

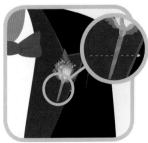

Pin to lapel.

No matter what your shape or style, there is an ensemble out there to make you look fantastic on your special day.

sheath dress
tall, slim-hipped

ball gown
hour-glass figure

mermaid cut
slender figure

empire waist
small-breasted, petite

strapless
toned arms

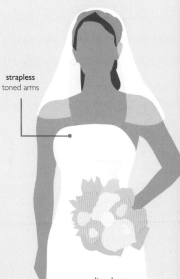

sweetheart neckline
large bustline

bateau neck
ample bosom

high collar
all body types

low v-neck
small bustline

a-line dress
flatters all body types

chapel
elegant event

watteau
informal; outdoors

cathedral
formal wedding

royal
state event

brush train
appropriate for
any wedding

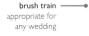

fingertip
any dress

waltz
dress without train

mantilla
simple gown

cathedral
formal gown

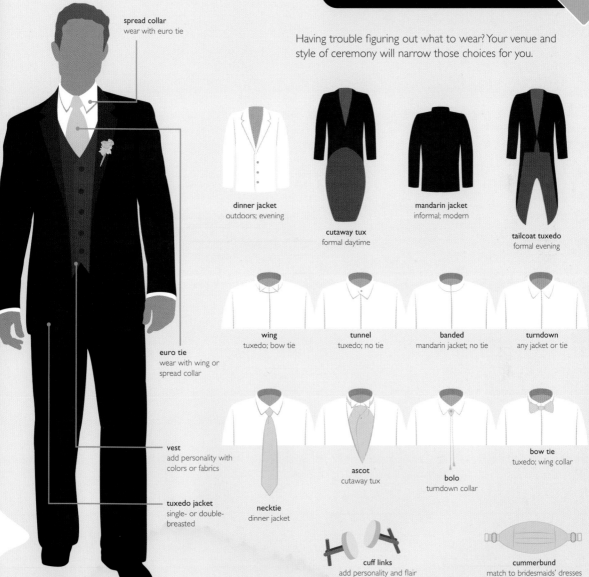

Having trouble figuring out what to wear? Your venue and style of ceremony will narrow those choices for you.

spread collar
wear with euro tie

euro tie
wear with wing or spread collar

vest
add personality with colors or fabrics

tuxedo jacket
single- or double-breasted

dinner jacket
outdoors; evening

cutaway tux
formal daytime

mandarin jacket
informal; modern

tailcoat tuxedo
formal evening

wing
tuxedo; bow tie

tunnel
tuxedo; no tie

banded
mandarin jacket; no tie

turndown
any jacket or tie

necktie
dinner jacket

ascot
cutaway tux

bolo
turndown collar

bow tie
tuxedo; wing collar

cuff links
add personality and flair

cummerbund
match to bridesmaids' dresses

zombie ceremony

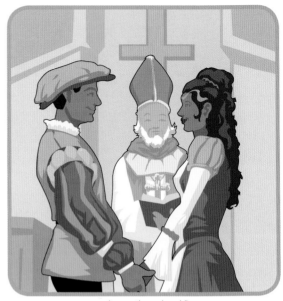

renaissance-themed wedding

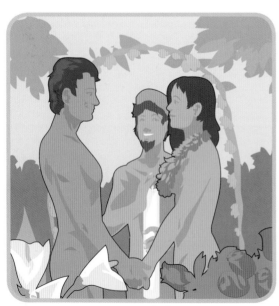

vows au naturel

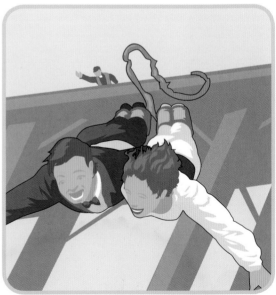

bungee bride

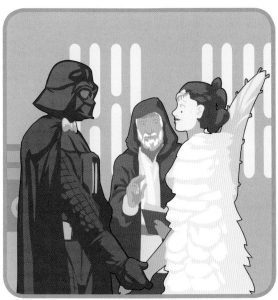

science-fiction nuptuals

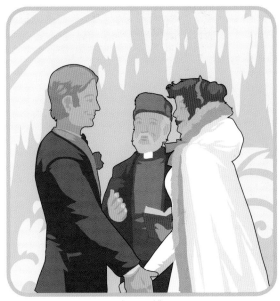

wintry wedding

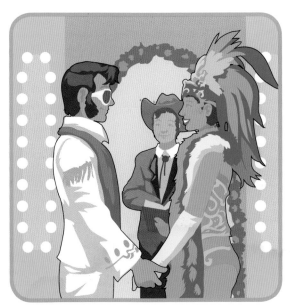

vegas vows

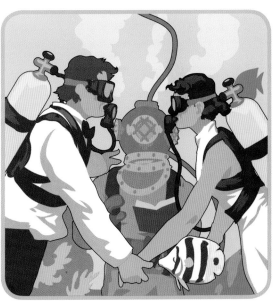

underwater union

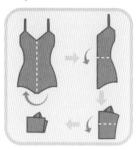
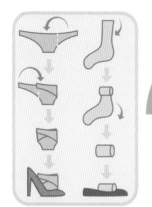
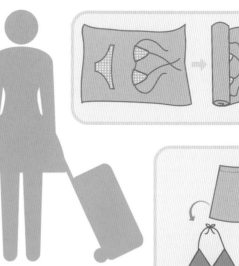
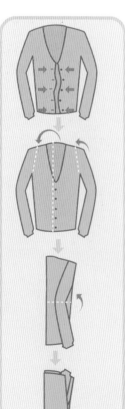
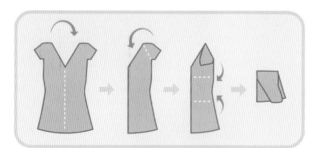
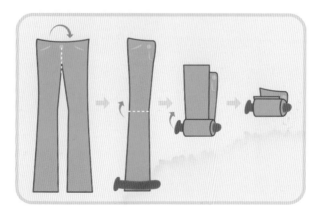
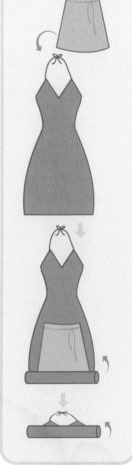

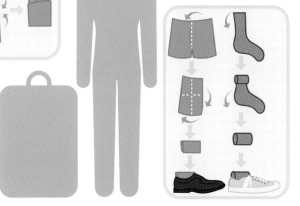

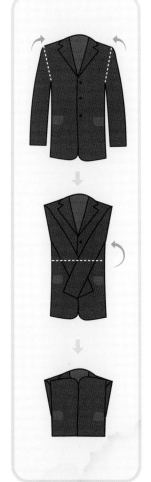

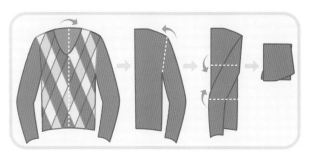

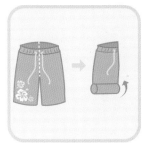

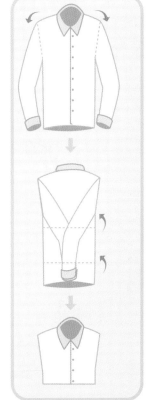

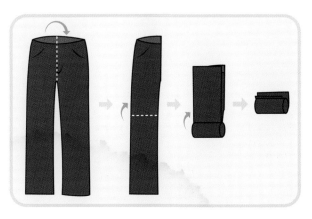

Try to spot Venus in the night sky. This bright planet shines a love light in the evening and morning.

Get dirty, then get clean, then get dirty again with sensual bath products.

Turn off that phone. You can get back to sexting later.

Close those drapes—you don't want to shock (or awe) the neighbors.

Serve up sensuous, sexy foods like fondue. Don't forget the bubbly!

Let pets frolic outside while you frolic indoors.

Live in a secluded spot? Lucky you! Pack a picnic basket full of naughty treats and head outdoors.

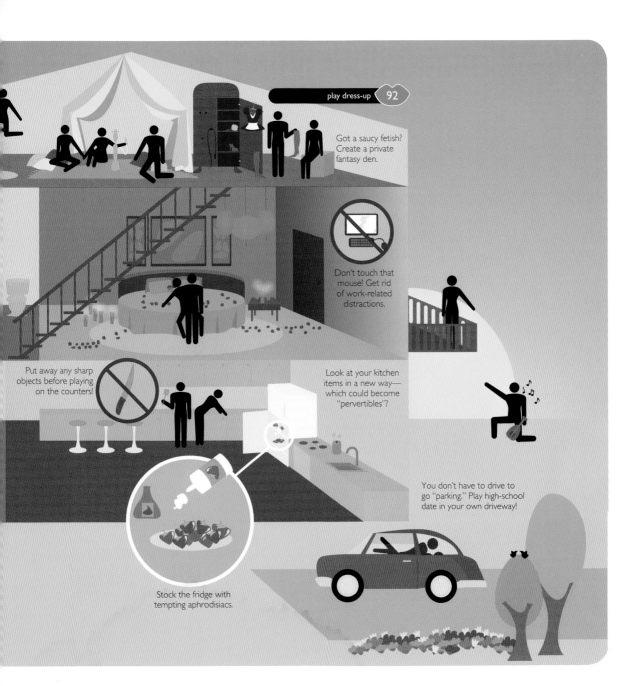

Got a saucy fetish? Create a private fantasy den.

Don't touch that mouse! Get rid of work-related distractions.

Put away any sharp objects before playing on the counters!

Look at your kitchen items in a new way— which could become "pervertibles"?

You don't have to drive to go "parking." Play high-school date in your own driveway!

Stock the fridge with tempting aphrodisiacs.

A lifelong relationship means a life of amazing memories. Keep the spark aflame every day by trying new things and never falling into a boring routine.

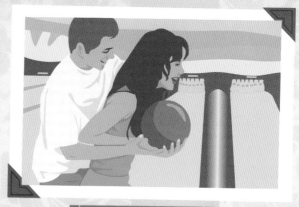

Develop a fun, goofy hobby you can enjoy as a team.

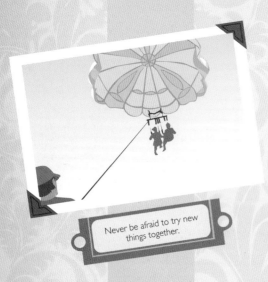

Never be afraid to try new things together.

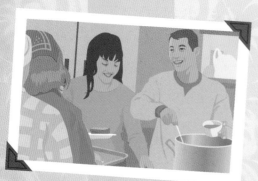

Helping out others is good for you and for the world.

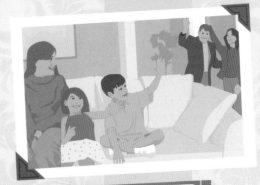

Happy parents know that kid-free date nights are essential.

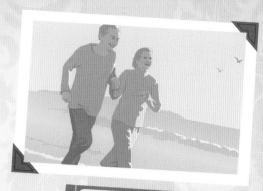

Stay healthy and
active together.

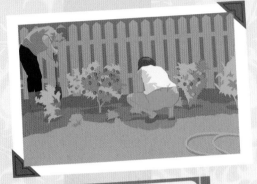

Home-improvement projects
are more fun when shared.

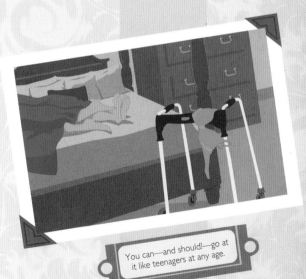

You can—and should!—go at
it like teenagers at any age.

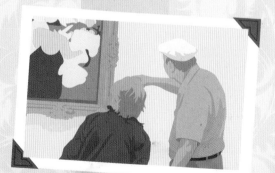

Stoke your passions
for art and culture.

tools

 love potion

 car

 raspberries

 candle

 tie

 mp3 player

 picnic basket

 moisturizer

 condom

 rope

 undies

 match

 nail file

 massage oil

 boutonniere greens

 breath mint

 cherry

 stewardess uniform

 barbershop quartet

 cuticle stick

 chopstick

 presents

 florist wire

 tip

 '70s dress

 wig

 old sheet

 clippers

 breakfast tray

 soothing aloe balm

 bouquet greenery

 pillow

 dog toy

 lipliner

 hair rollers

 scissors

 doggy treat

 apology bouquet

 florist tape

 garter belt

 credit card

 lipstick

 talcum powder

 '70s duds

 eyelid-primer brush

 comb

 pool table

 notepad

 bra

 plane with banner

 sugar

 surprise breakfast

 satin ribbon

 bottled beer

 hair-removal wax

 yoga mat

 lip balm

 concert flyer

 long-stem roses

 pool cue

 eyelid primer

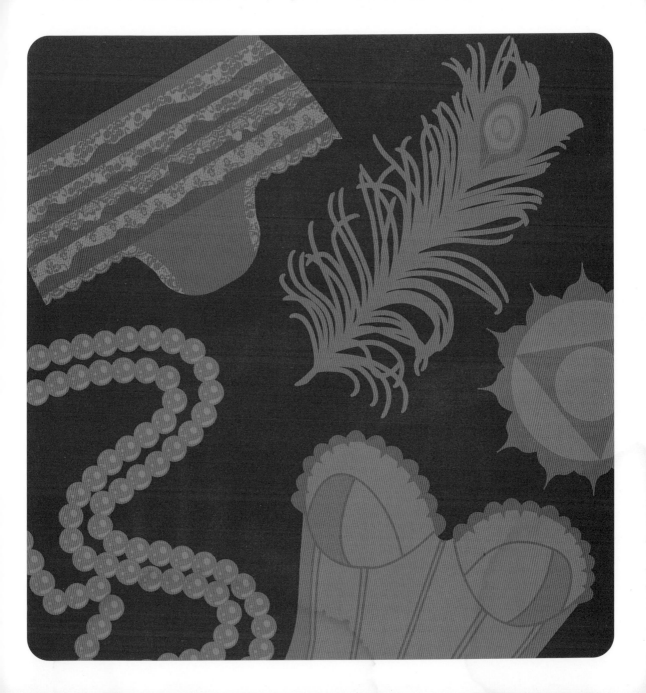

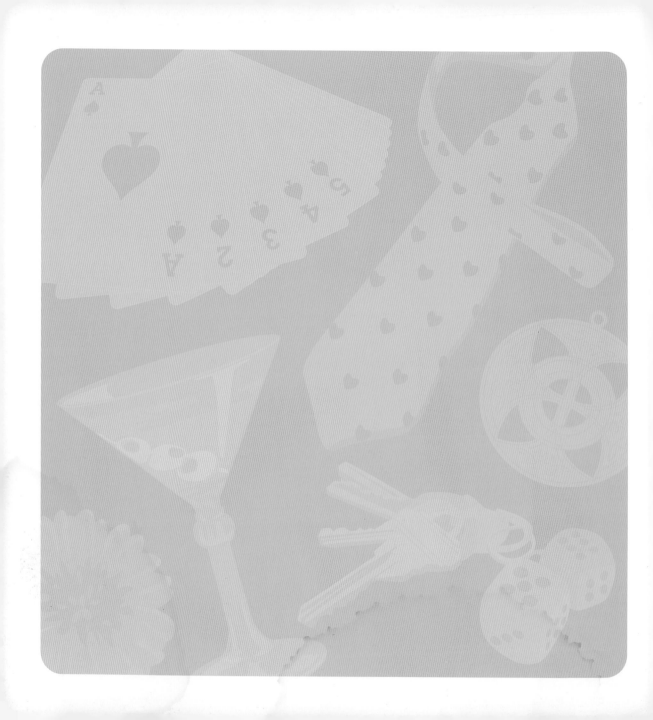

parchment paper

bowl

lip gloss

sharp knife

bow tie

keys

video camera

blender

waxing strips

note paper

cosmetic scissors

tweezers

safety pin

smoky eyeshadow

little black book

licorice

pencil

notebook

diamond ring

hair clips

blindfold

briefcase

seductive underpinnings

suit

taxi

bath towel

butter knife

corset lace

pen

eyeshadow brush

eyeliner

diva heels

banana

ice cubes

lip brush

cotton swab

blow dryer

nail clippers

corset

pins

television

napkin

cell phone

hair spray

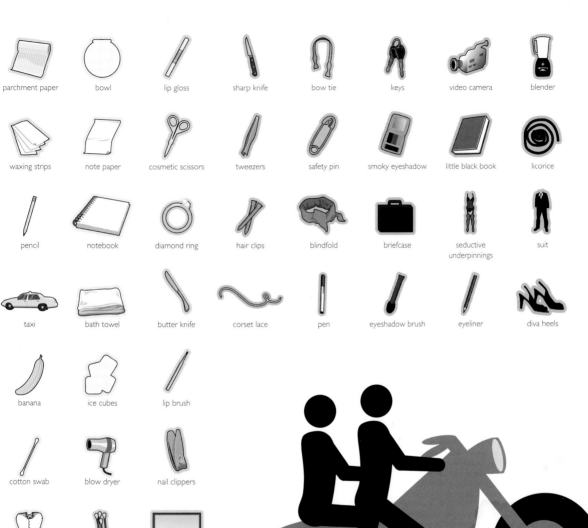

index

45

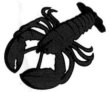

57

67

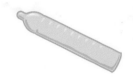

85

150

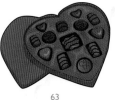

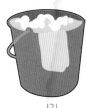

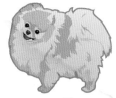

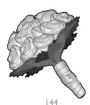

120

47

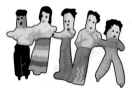

1

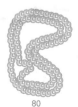

80

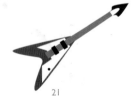

21

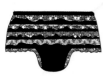

73

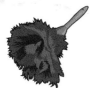

102

133

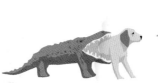

131

96

show me who

WELDON OWEN INC.

CEO, President Terry Newell

VP, Sales and
New Business Development Amy Kaneko

VP, Publisher Roger Shaw

Creative Director Kelly Booth

Executive Editor Mariah Bear

Editor Lucie Parker

Project Editor Frances Reade

Production Editor Emelie Griffin

Art Director Marisa Kwek

Senior Designer Stephanie Tang

Designers Delbarr Moradi, Meghan Hildebrand

Illustration Coordinators
Conor Buckley, Sheila Masson

Production Director Chris Hemesath

Production Manager Michelle Duggan

Production Coordinator Charles Mathews

Color Manager Teri Bell

weldon**owen**

415 Jackson Street, Suite 200
San Francisco, CA 94111
Telephone: 415 291 0100
Fax: 415 291 8841

www.wopublishing.com

Weldon Owen is a division of
BONNIER

Library of Congress data is on file with the
Publisher.

ISBN: 978-1-61628-220-2

10 9 8 7 6 5 4 3 2

Printed in China by 1010 Printing Ltd.

Special thanks to:

Storyboarders
Sarah Duncan, Kenneth Holland, Jonathan Shariat,
Jamie Spinello, Brandi Valenza

Illustration specialists
Hayden Foell, Raymond Larrett, Jamie Spinello,
Ross Sublett

Editorial and research support team
Chug Pub, Kat Engh, Michael Alexander Eros, Justin
Goers, Susan Jonaitis, Marisa Solis, Stefanos Tiziano

A **Show Me Now** Book.
Show Me Now is a trademark
of Weldon Owen Inc.
www.showmenow.com

ILLUSTRATION CREDITS The artwork in this book
was a true team effort. We are happy to thank and
acknowledge our illustrators.

Front Cover: **Christine Meighan:** peacock feather
Jamie Spinello: lingerie **Bryon Thompson:** condom, whip
Gabhor Utomo: Champagne

Back Cover: **Juan Calle (Liberum Donum):** pole dance
Jamie Spinello: sexy stranger, key-party attendees

Key bg=background, ex=extra art

Steve Baletsa: 72 **Kelly Booth:** 33 **Juan Calle (Liberum
Donum):** 14, 24–25, 29, 35, 46, 54–55, 68–69, 79,
83–84, 87–90, 94–96, 103–104, 115–116, 121, 126, 148
Sarah Duncan: 32, 34, 129–130 **Hayden Foell:** 55 ex,
56–57, 81–82, 83 ex, 86, 100–102, 133 **Britt Hanson:**
4–7, 15–23, 36–37, 50–53, 64–67, 92–93, 103 bg,
105–108, 111, 113–114, 124, 127–128, 131 bg, 140 bg,
149–151 **Jessica Henry:** 49, 119 **Pilar Erika Johnson:**
42–44 **Vic Kulihin:** 99 **Raymond Larrett:** 120, 122

Christine Meighan: 12, 48, 58–60, 78, 80, 109, 112,
140–141 **Jamie Spinello:** 73, 75, 97, 125, 132 **Ross
Sublett:** 70–71, 104 bg **Bryon Thompson:** 45, 85, 91,
146–147 **Gabhor Utomo:** 1–3, 27–28, 30, 38–41, 62,
77, 111 bg, 118, 125 ex, 131,132 ex, 136–139, 152
Tina Cash Walsh: 8–11, 26, 31, 47, 61, 63, 74, 76, 98,
117, 123, 134–135, 142–143 **Mary Zins:** 13, 110, 123,
144–145

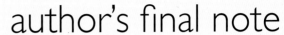

author's final note

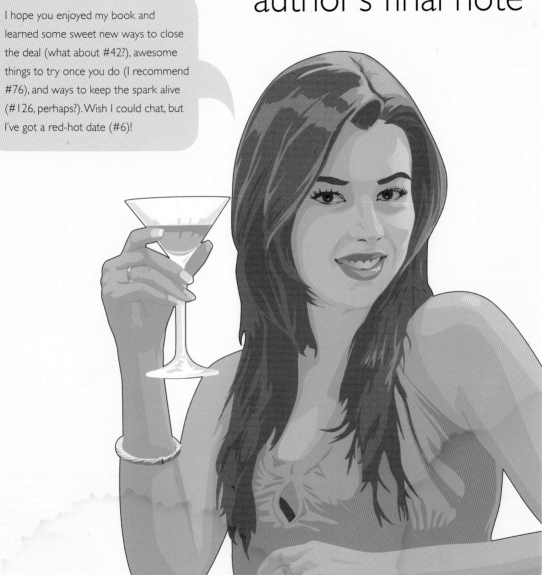

I hope you enjoyed my book and learned some sweet new ways to close the deal (what about #42?), awesome things to try once you do (I recommend #76), and ways to keep the spark alive (#126, perhaps?). Wish I could chat, but I've got a red-hot date (#6)!

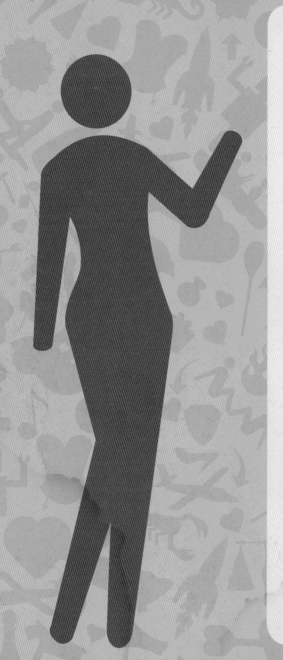

hey, sailor!

Is there something romantic that you think should have been included in this book? Do you have a sexy or sweet skill that you want to share with the rest of the world? Is there something we didn't get quite right? If so, we want to know all about it!

We love hearing from our highly talented readers. Send us your ideas, feedback, or even photos or video of you demonstrating your skills (please, nothing we'd be too embarrassed to show our moms), and you could be featured in the next Show Me Now book.

We can't wait to hear from you!

www.showmenow.com

ATTN: SHOW ME TEAM
Weldon Owen Inc.
415 Jackson Street
San Francisco, California 94111